Notes for the
DRCOG

Notes for the DRCOG

Peter Kaye
MA MB BChir MRCP MRCGP DRCOG
Consultant in Continuing Care, Northampton

Second edition

CHURCHILL LIVINGSTONE
EDINBURGH LONDON MELBOURNE AND NEW YORK 1988

CHURCHILL LIVINGSTONE
Medical Division of Longman Group UK Limited

Distributed in the United States of America by Churchill
Livingstone Inc., 1560 Broadway, New York,
N.Y. 10036, and by associated companies, branches
and representatives throughout the world.

First published 1983
Second edition 1983
Reprinted 1989

ISBN 0-443-03785-X

British Library Cataloguing in Publication Data
Kaye, Peter, 1953–
  Notes for the DRCOG. — 2nd ed.
  1. Gynaecology — Examinations, questions, etc.   2. Obstetrics —
  Examinations, questions, etc.
  I. Title
  618'.076   RG111

Library of Congress Cataloging in Publication Data
Kaye, Peter.
  Notes for the DRCOG.

  Includes index.
  1. Gynecology — Examinations, questions, etc. 2. Obstetrics —
  Examinations, questions, etc. 3. Neonatology — Examinations,
  questions, etc. I. Title. [DNLM: 1. Gynecology — examination
  questions. 2. Neonatology — examination questions.
  3. Obstetrics — examination questions.   WP 18 K23n]
  RG111.K39   1988   618   87-15118

Printed in Great Britain at The Bath Press, Avon.

Preface to the Second Edition

This book is mainly intended for GP trainees revising for the DRCOG, but final year students might also find it useful. The wide margin is for additional notes. It aims to provide up-to-date information on practical management problems. For the sake of brevity only one acceptable method of management is usually outlined, and there are a lot of abbreviations used, all of which are explained in a glossary at the end of the book.

This edition has been extensively revised. There have been recent advances in obstetric practice in several areas. New sections have been included on: chorionic villus biopsy; Pre-natal diagnosis; Maternal serum AFP screening; In vitro fertilization; The ultrasound scan; An antenatal checklist; AIDS.

New sections have also been added on Antiprogesterones, the Premenstrual syndrome, colposcopy and ablative therapy, hysterectomy, the contraceptive sponge, spermicides, thyroid disease in pregnancy, rare medical conditions in pregnancy, drugs in pregnancy, vacuum extraction, the transcutaneous nerve stimulator, and puerperal depression.

The following sections have been extensively revised or rewritten: Hirsutism; Infertility; Cervical smears; The combined pill; Research in contraception; Maternal mortality; Preconception clinics; Minor symptoms in pregnancy; Diabetes; Rhesus disease; Home deliveries.

I am very grateful to the following for their helpful comments: Mr Ed. Shaxted, Consultant Obstetrician; Dr Charles Fox, Consultant Physician; Dr Nick Griffin, Consultant Paediatrician; Dr Simon Thompson, General Practitioner; and to Sheila Kitzinger for her help with the section on Alternative Methods of Childbirth.

I am also very grateful to the many people who took the trouble to write to me with suggestions and comments. I would again welcome comments about the second edition via the publishers.

Northampton, 1988   P K

Contents

Gynaecology

History   1. *The complaint*
2. *Date of LMP* and cycle (e.g. 5/28).

— pain (during or preceding)
— heaviness (clots? how many tampons?)
— bleeding (between periods, postcoital)
— age of menarche

3. *Parity*. Detailed obstetric history. Terminations
4. *Discharge* (colour, duration, itch, soreness, partner)
5. *Abdomen* (pain, bowels, dysuria, stress or urge incontinence)
6. *Intercourse* (pain, problems) contraception
7. *Past history*. Date of last smear. Previous curettage, cone biopsy, cryocautery, laparoscopy or general surgery
8. *Emotional problems* (Family and social history)

Examination   1. General appearance (stature, breasts, hirsutism)
2. Palpate the abdomen (laparoscopy scars, tenderness, lumps)
3. Inspect the vulva (redness, atrophy, urethral discharge, Bartholin's cyst, warts, ulceration or carcinoma)
4. Pass a speculum, inspect the cervix and take a smear. Take a high vaginal swab (HVS) of any vaginal discharge and endocervical and urethral swabs if gonorrhoea is suspected.
5. Bimanual examination. Tenderness on moving the cervix occurs in salpingitis and ectopic pregnancy. Note whether the os is small and nulliparous or patulous and multiparous. Note whether the uterus is anteverted, axial or retroverted and whether it is enlarged (pregnancy or fibroids). Palpate the adnexae for tenderness or lumps (when ultrasound and/or laparoscopy may be necessary for diagnosis).

The menstrual cycle   1. *Bleeding* occurs because corpus luteal function fades, oestrogen and progesterone levels fall (and FSH rises) and the unsupported endometrium sloughs. The average blood loss is 60 ml and clotting is prevented by endometrial fibrinolysins.
2. The rising FSH stimulates ovarian follicles (*follicular phase*) one of which develops and secretes oestrogen. The oestrogen causes proliferation of the ducts in the breast and endometrium (*proliferative phase*) and increases cervical mucus and the glycogen content of vaginal squames.
3. The rising oestrogen at a critical level causes an LH surge, an ovum is released from the ovary and the corpus luteum is formed.

4. During the second half of the cycle (*luteal phase*) the corpus luteum secretes both oestrogen and progesterone, which causes an elevation in temperature (0.5°C), secretory changes in the breast and endometrium (*secretory phase*) and a drying of cervical mucus.

5. *Implantation* of a fertilized ovum results in HCG secretion by the trophoblast. This has anLH — like action and supports the corpus luteum, which continues to secrete oestrogen and progesterone, maintaining the endometrium until the placenta takes over (12 weeks).

Ovulation can be demonstrated by:

— ovulatory cascade of cervical mucus (Billings method)
— raised body temperature (+0.25−0.5°C)
— raised serum progesterone on day 21 (or urine pregnandiol)
— endometrial biopsy (showing secretory changes in the luteal phase of the cycle)

Oestrogens   Oestradiol 17β is synthesized from cholesterol and metabolized to oestrone and oestriol. They are excreted in the urine and can be measured (e.g. during Pergonal therapy). Synthetic preparations are used therapeutically (ethinyloestradiol and stilboestrol). Premarin is a mixture of conjugated oestrogens derived from pregnant mares' urine. Oestrogens have the following actions:

— pituitary inhibition
— secondary sexual development
— fusion of the epiphyses
— myometrial hypertrophy
— endometrial hyperplasia (hence withdrawal bleeds)
— increased cervical mucus
— vaginal cornification (increased squames)
— sodium retention
— tendency to thrombosis

They are *used* in:

1. The Combined Pill
2. Hormone replacement after the menopause, for atrophic vaginitis or hot flushes, or in ovarian dysgenesis, e.g. ethinyloestradiol 20 µg daily. If used for a long period, a progestagen should be added because of the risk of endometrial carcinoma.
3. Cancer. Stilboestrol is less potent than ethinyloestradiol and is used to treat carcinoma of the prostate (1 mg daily).

Progestagens   Progesterone is produced by the corpus luteum and placenta and metabolized in the liver to pregnanediol. Progesterone assay is used to confirm ovulation. Progesterone has the following actions:

— pituitary inhibition

— raised body temperature (0.5°C)
— secretory changes (breast, uterus)
— decreased cervical mucus
— uterine contractions (slow)
— maintainance of pregnancy

Synthetic preparations are used therapeutically. They are *classified* into:

1. Natural derivatives — e.g. hydroxyprogesterone 250 mg i.m. twice weekly for early habitual abortions and long-acting medroxyprogesterone (Depo-Provera) 150 mg i.m. for contraception.
2. Testosterone derivatives — e.g. norethisterone (Primolut N) 5 mg t.d.s. used for dysfunctional uterine bleeding. It is metabolised to testosterone and is therefore not used to treat habitual abortion.
3. Stereo-isomers of progesterone — e.g. dydrogesterone (Duphaston) 10 mg b.d.

Progesterones are also used in the Combined Pill, and high-dose progesterone (e.g. medroxyprogesterone 250 mg daily) is used to palliate advanced uterine carcinoma.

Antiprogesterones Useful antagonists have been developed to several of the 5 steroid hormones:

oestrogens   — clomiphene, tamoxifen
androgens   — cyproterone
progesterones   —
mineralocorticoids — spironolactone
glucocorticoids   —

Antiprogesterones are being developed which are not androgenic and do not interfere with the synthesis of adrenal steroids. Progesterone is a key hormone in establishing and maintaining pregnancy. An antiprogesterone would therefore:

— induce menstruation (given in luteal phase)
— prevent implantation (given day 24–26)
— induce abortion (given in early pregnancy)

Antiprogesterones may offer new therapeutic possibilities for contraception and therapeutic abortion.

Primary amenorrhoea Most girls have their first period before the age of 16. Other signs of puberty normally precede menstruation by about a year and if longer than 2 years then an absent vagina or an imperforate hymen is likely. No breast development by the age of 14 merits investigations:

— breast growth (8.5–13 years)
— pubic hair
— axillary hair

— growth spurt
— menarche

*Primary amenorrhoea is best classified according to whether these
secondary sexual characteristics are present, absent or heterosexual.*

1. Present
— imperforate hymen
— absent vagina (XX) ± uterus
— absent vagina (XY — i.e. testicular feminization)

If the vagina seems absent, perform a PRA mass anteriorly
suggests haematocolpos due to a vaginal septum.

If the vagina is absent chromosomal analysis is necessary. If
XX, an IVU is important because renal anomalies are commonly
associated.

An artificial vagina is most simply fashioned by forming an
external perineal pouch (Williams's operation) which is enlarged
initially with dilators.

If laparoscopy reveals a normal uterus then an internal vagina
can be constructed (McIndoe–Read operation).

2. Absent or poor
— Constitutional
— Hypothalamic (Kallman's syndrome)
— Pituitary tumour
— Ovarian dysgenesis (XO or XX)
— Systemic or endocrine disease

Most cases are constitutional and there is usually a family
history of late puberty in one parent to aid diagnosis.

If the girl is short (under 1.47 m — 4 foot 10 inches), Turner's
syndrome (XO) must always be considered (poor growth is due
to loss of chromosomal material). In pure gonadal dysgenesis
(XX) there are no sex hormones produced so the patient is tall
(no epiphyseal fusion) and FSH will be high.

After 16 (or before if breast development, height or weight
are delayed by more than 2 years) other causes must be excluded.
Careful history and examination usually reveals any systemic
ill-health (coeliac disease, renal tubular acidosis and anorexia
nervosa can be overlooked). Serum thyroxine must always be
estimated and pituitary tumours (usually craniopharyngioma)
excluded by skull X-rays and gonadotrophin assays. Hyperprolactinaemia can rarely present with primary amenorrhoea.
Kallman's syndrome consists of anosmia and specific failure to
secrete FSH and LH.

3. Signs of virilization
These include hirsutism, cliteromegaly, muscular development;
consider:

— Intersex (e.g. XY with cryptorchidism and hypogonadism)
— Congenital adrenal hyperplasia (CAH)
— Tumour (adrenal or ovary)

Examine the genitalia for normality and the labia and groins for lumps (testes) and abdomen for large ovarian mass. Chromosomal analysis and hormone assays will be essential in every case and may lead to other tests (laparoscopy, adrenal scan).

Imperforate hymen
— breast and pubic hair normal
— periodic lower abdominal pain
— urinary hesitancy and retention
— bulging bluish membrane (may be high and not visible)
— abdominal mass
— PR mass anteriorly (haematocolpos)

The membrane is incised under sterile conditions.

Testicular feminization
XY with normal testes but androgen insensitivity, hence the female phenotype develops, but female internal organs are absent due to Mullerian Inhibitory Factor. The appearances are of a normal girl, often attractive, with good breast development, but there is:

— no sexual hair
— short blind vagina
— absent uterus
— testes (intra-abdominal, inguinal, labial)
— high (i.e. male) testosterone levels
— XY karyotype

Examination reveals an absent vagina and cervix. Diagnosis is by chromosomal analysis and serum testosterone. Orchidectomy is indicated in case of malignant change. Oestrogen replacement maintains breast development and prevents hot flushes.

Turner's syndrome
Ovarian dygenesis (streak ovaries) with other abnormalities due to loss of chromosomal material (XO). A combination of short stature and absent secondary sexual characteristics is highly suggestive of Turner's syndrome. The other features may or may not be present:

— webbed neck
— widely spaced nipples
— wide carrying-angle at elbow
— short metatarsals
— coarctation of the aorta.

Turner's syndrome is diagnosed by chromosomal analysis (XO). It is treated with cyclical ethinyloestradiol 0.02 mg (three weeks in four) with norethisterone 5 mg daily during the third week. This causes breast development and cyclical bleeding and can be continued unchanged into adult life. It is replacement therapy and does not cause further stunting of growth.

Puberty   1. The physical signs of puberty are:

— breast growth (average 11 years)
— pubic hair
— axillary hair
— growth spurt
— menstruation (average 13 years)

The changes occur due to hypothalamic maturation and also due to the synthesis (from adrenal precursors) of oestrogens in fat — the average *weight* of menarche is 47 kg.

2. Intersex may first be recognized at puberty, either because of primary amenorrhoea due to testicular feminization (XY) or a mild form of CAH (XX) or because the 'girl' (in fact XY with cryptorchidism and hypospadias) develops clitoromegaly and a deep voice due to rising testosterone levels. Generally it is best to try to retain the sex to which the patient has adjusted psychologically.

3. Puberty may be delayed (see primary amenorrhoea).

4. Precocious puberty is defined as breast development before the age of 8 or periods before the age of 10. Pregnancy has been recorded at the age of 5.

The possibilities are:

— constitutional
— hypothalamic tumour (CT scan) and postencephalitis
— ovarian tumour (laparoscopy)
— adrenal tumour (also virilized; raised oxo-steroids)

Tumours must be excluded. Medroxyprogesterone or the anti-gonadotrophin danazol can prevent menstruation and stunting of growth due to premature fusion of the epiphyses.

5. The first cycles are usually anovular, and heavy dysfunctional bleeding can occur. The girl and her mother can be reassured that it usually settles down after 3 or 4 cycles. (If it does not, EUA is important to exclude an ovarian tumour.) Norethisterone 5 mg b.d. can be given for the week before the period. Iron is rarely necessary. A rare cause in some countries is endometrial tuberculosis diagnosed by curettage.

Dysmenorrhoea   1. Primary dysmenorrhoea means colicky menstrual cramps that occurs on Day 1 of the period, with pain in the suprapubic region, low back and groins. The pain only occurs in ovulatory cycles, presumably because a raised progesterone is necessary to produce the high prostaglandin levels found in the menstrual fluid in these girls. Periods usually become painful soon after puberty once the cycles become ovulatory. Nausea, diarrhoea and flushing can occur. It is nearly always cured by childbirth. Reassurance and explanation are important. There are three main approaches to treatment:

a) Analgesics and antispasmodics, e.g. hyoscine (Buscopan) 20 mg q.d.s.

b) Prostaglandin inhibitors, e.g. mefenamic acid (Ponstan) 500 mg q.d.s.
c) The Combined Pill to inhibit ovulation

Cervical dilatation or presacral neurectomy are now very rarely used.

2. Secondary or congestive dysmenorrhoea occurs in middle-aged women with endometriosis or chronic salpingitis and may be an indication for laparoscopy. The pain usually starts several days before the period, is constant rather than colicky and is often associated with back pain, deep dyspareunia and some-times menorrhagia. When no pathology is found it is ascribed to pelvic congestion and the possibility of psychosexual problems is considered.

Premenstrual Syndrome (PMS)

Premenstrual syndrome (PMS) is an important condition and has been used in court as a successful defence against murder. PMS was described in 1931 by Frank, who ascribed the symptoms to excess oestrogen and treated women with oopho-rectomy. 'Medical oophorectomy' with a GnRH agonist has also been shown experimentally to alleviate the symptoms (long-acting GnRH agonists block rather than stimulate the pituitary).

The pathophysiology of PMS is not understood but the symptom complex and mood changes suggest hypothalamic neurotransmitters are involved. The symptoms of PMS include:

— Bloating, oedema (fluid retention)
— Headaches
— Breast swelling and pain
— Change in bowel habit
— Mood changes and irritability
— Depression (affecting sleep, sex, appetite, concentration)

The symptoms recur in the late luteal phase of the cycle, are often more severe with prolonged intermenstrual intervals, regress with the onset of menstrual bleeding and are associated with at least one symptom-free week following menstruation. PMS is more common with age, parity, stress and lack of exer-cise. Differential diagnosis includes dysmenorrhoea, endo-metriosis, psychological disorders and psychosexual disorders.

Management involves a detailed history (menstrual, obstetric, contraceptive and sexual) and examination to exclude disease and to reassure. With time and patience symptoms can nearly always be considerably improved. Ongoing support is important and a menstrual chart to document symptoms can be useful. Treatment is empirical and in all studies the placebo effect has been high. The following are thought to help:

— Exercise and improved fitness
— Diet (small, frequent meals, roughage, protein, low sugar, low salt)
— Pyridoxine 100 mg daily

For particular symptoms treat the most severe first:

— Mefanamic acid 500 mg t.i.d. (headache)
— Spironolactone 100 mg daily, days 18–28 (fluid retention)
— Dydrogesterone 10 mg BD days 12–26 (psychological symptoms)
— Bromocryptine 5 mg nocte (mastalgia)

Dydrogesterone (Duphaston) has been shown to be more effective than placebo. In severe PMS Danazol 200 mg daily may be justified where other measures have failed.

Heavy periods   *Menorrhagia* means heavy regular periods. It is a symptom which suggests that local lesions are unlikely. A menstrual calendar may be useful. Severity is deduced clinically from:

— clots
— towels as well as tampons
— more than 10 days
— socially inconvenienced
— anaemia

Causes   The causes are:

1. Dysfunctional bleeding
2. IUCD
3. Fibroids or adenomyosis
4. Hypothyroidism
5. Clotting disorders

Management   1. *Dysfunctional bleeding* usually occurs in women over 35. It eventually resolves without treatment. Perform a VE to exclude fibroids or tenderness (adenomyosis or salpingitis).
There are two types of dysfunctional bleeding:

a) *Ovulatory and regular* — heavy bleeding is due to a poor luteal phase. When bleeding is regular it is safe to try hormones. Norethisterone 5–10 mg daily for the last 10 days of the cycle often decreases blood loss. A high progesterone pill can be used instead, e.g. Anovlar (ethinyloestradiol 50 μg, norethisterone 4 mg). Alternatively a prostaglandin inhibitor, e.g. flurbiprofen (Froben) 100 mg t.d.s. often decreases blood loss.

b) *Anovular and chaotic*. Typically the persistently high oestrogen levels cause 6–8 weeks amenorrhoea followed by heavy prolonged bleeding. The pattern is irregular and currettage is indicated to exclude pathology (incomplete abortion, polyp, carcinoma).
   Curettage often cures the problem. If the problem recurs norethisterone or Anovlar can be used, then stopped after 6 months to see if spontaneous cure has occurred.
   Hysterectomy may be considered in a woman who has completed her family.

2. The IUCD often causes heavy periods. The woman may prefer to try a smaller device (e.g. Multiload) or use another method of contraception.

Alternatively Froben can be used to decrease blood loss. Tranexamic acid is also effective. This is an anti-fibrinolytic which inhibits uterine fibrinolysins and decreases bleeding. It may cause nausea and is contraindicated with a history of thrombosis.

3. Fibroids, adenomyosis (tender bulky uterus) or chronic salpingitis can cause heavy periods. There are usually other symptoms. Perform VE and consider laparoscopy.

4. Hypothyroidism can present (rarely) with menorrhagia. Other features are lethargy, cold intolerance, myalgia, deafness, carpal tunnel syndrome, dry skin and hair and puffy eyelids. Bradycardia usually occurs but the pulse rate may be normal if menorrhagia has caused anaemia. Diagnosis is by a low serum thyroxine and raised TSH. Thyroxine replacement cures the problem.

5. Thrombocytopenia or Von Willebrand's disease can present (very rarely) with menorrhagia. If suspected (from bruising, bleeding, or family history) measure:

— platelet count
— prothrombin time
— KPTT

Von Willebrand's disease is dominantly inherited so there should be a family history. The above tests can all be normal and the diagnosis is made on low Factor VIII levels (both coagulant and antigenic) and abnormal platelet aggregation (negative with ristocetin). Bleeding can be treated with fresh frozen plasma, but hysterectomy is usually necessary.

Intermenstrual bleeding

Non-menstrual bleeding suggests a carcinoma until proved otherwise. The bleeding may be postcoital, intermenstrual or postmenopausal. The possible causes are:

— abortion or ectopic
— dysfunctional, POP, IUCD
— vaginitis, endometritis
— cervical erosion
— polyp
— carcinoma

Management

1. Always consider pregnancy. Irregular bleeding with abdominal pains may be an indication for laparoscopy to exclude an ectopic pregnancy. Persistent irregular bleeding 6 weeks after an abortion suggests an incomplete abortion (or rarely choriocarcinoma).

2. A woman is allowed 1 or 2 cycles with intermenstrual bleeding if she has just started using the POP (breakthrough

bleeds) or the IUCD. If she is having chaotic dysfunctional cycles curettage is indicated and usually cures the problem.

3. Examine the vulva, vagina, cervix and uterus, take a smear and refer for a diagnostic curettage. Even if a post-menopausal woman has obvious atrophic vaginitis to explain the bleeding, curettage is mandatory to exclude an endometrial carcinoma. If a postmenopausal woman who is not on hormone replacement therapy (HRT) is having irregular bleeding and curettings show proliferative changes due to oestrogens then a functioning granulosa cell tumour (usually small) of the ovary is present and BSO and hysterectomy would be performed.

Secondary amenorrhoea   This is the cessation of periods for more than 6 months between the ages of 16–40, having excluded pregnancy.

99% are due to endocrine causes and all are treatable except premature ovarian failure.

Always consider:

— pregnancy
— hypothalamic (weight loss, stress) — 45%
— hypothalamic but responding to clomiphene — 20%
— hyperprolactinaemia — 20%
— premature ovarian failure — 10%
— polycystic ovary syndrome (POS) — 4%
— hypothyroidism — 1%

Rare causes are hypopituitarism, Cushing's syndrome, virilizing tumours, Turner's mosaicism (XO/XX) when a few periods can occur before presenting as secondary amenorrhoea and uterine occlusion due to tuberculosis or fibrosis following traumatic curettage — *Aschermann's syndrome.*

N.B. Post-pill amenorrhoea is best considered to be secondary amenorrhoea that has been masked by regular withdrawal bleeds. It should be investigated, but usually no abnormality is found and it virtually always responds to clomiphene.

Management   1. Ask about:

— possibility of pregnancy
— weight loss, emotional upset
— previous menstrual pattern
— pill or other drugs.
— galactorrhoea
— hot flushes
— hirsutism (may be well disguised)
— general health (especially thyroid symptoms)

2. Examine for hirsutism or signs of thyroid disorder. VE to exclude pregnancy and assess the size of the ovaries. Ultrasound scan may be necessary to exclude pregnancy.

3. If the woman is obese and hirsute, she is usually assumed

to have polycystic ovary syndrome (POS). A serum testosterone is measured to exclude virilizing tumours (when it would be high) and clomiphene will induce ovulation if fertility is required.

4. If the woman is well and pregnancy has been excluded the progesterone provacation test is safe. Norethisterone 5 mg b.d. is given for 1 week. If a withdrawal bleed occurs then the woman must be well oestrogenized and is simply having anovular cycles. Both menstruation and fertility will return with clomiphene.

This condition is said to be due to a 'cycle initiation defect' with a presumed inability of the hypothalamus to initiate normal follicular development that will procede to ovulation. (In POS oestrogen levels are high and progesterone would also cause a withdrawal bleed.)

5. If progesterone fails to cause a withdrawal bleed then hormone assays are necessary.

— FSH (high in ovarian failure)
— prolactin
— free thyroxine index

6. If the woman is not hirsute and these hormone assays are normal the cause is hypothalamic due to weight loss or stress.

Losing more than 10 kg (unless the woman is already obese) tends to cause amenorrhoea and the woman need not necessarily have anorexia nervosa. Stress such as travel or a new job may cause amenorrhoea.

Both these problems may resolve and periods will return. Clomiphene is ineffective (because it cannot cause GnRH to rise). Pergonal will induce ovulation if immediate fertility is required but oestrogen levels need to be monitored. It is better to persuade the woman to regain weight, when periods and fertility will return.

7. In premature ovarian failure (high FSH) fertility cannot be restored and only HRT can be offered.

The other conditions are treatable but treatment can often be delayed until fertility is desired.

8. Meanwhile contraception is still necessary because the problem may resolve (weight loss, stress) or because sporadic ovulation may occur (POS and cycle initiation defect).

The Combined Pill can be safely used (and is also useful because in many of these conditions the woman is under-oestrogenized.)

In hyperprolactinaemia the pill was thought to cause enlargement of the pituitary tumour, but recent evidence suggests that the pill is safe if taken with bromocriptine.

Hyperprolactinaemia

High prolactin levels (above 4000 μu/ml) inhibit FSH and LH. The features are:

— amenorrhoea

— galactorrhoea (25%)
— pituitary tumour (40%)

If a tumour is not demonstrated by tomography and CT scan the cause is assumed to be a micro-adenoma. Prolactin levels do not vary with the menstrual cycle but are elevated by stress hence moderate elevation is common. The assay should always be repeated if the level is high. Drugs that are dopamine antagonists (phenothiazines, haloperidol, methyldopa, cimetidine, metoclopramide) will elevate prolactin, as will hypothyroidism. These must be excluded.

Treatment is with bromocryptine, a central dopamine agonist, which restores prolactin levels to normal almost immediately. Side-effects of nausea and postural hypotension are common so start with 2.5 mg after supper, gradually increasing to 5 mg t.d.s.

If there is a pituitary tumour, the treatment of choice is a selective excision via a transphenoidal approach which does not cause later hypopituitarism. If the woman gets pregnant on bromocriptine, visual fields are monitored because a pituitary tumour can enlarge in pregnancy. If the tumour does start to enlarge, bromocriptine should be continued throughout the pregnancy.

Galactorrhoea with normal periods cannot be due to hyperprolactinaemia and is usually due to repeated stimulation of the nipples, often sexual.

Polycystic ovary syndrome (POS)

— obesity (increased conversion of androgens to oestrogens), hence
— low FSH
— high LH (possibly due to persistently high oestrogens) hence
— multiple lutein cysts, producing
— androstendione (a 17 oxo-steroid), hence
— hirsutism
— oligomenorrhoea or amenorrhoea

Clinically an obese woman with amenorrhoea and hirsutism is initially assumed to have POS. It is diagnosed by laparoscopy. Increased urinary oxo-steroids and LH and a high LH/FSH ratio are typical. It is now recognized that a substantial number have secondary amenorrhoea without hirsutism or obesity. Plasma testosterone is normal, and useful to exclude virilizing tumours.

Clomiphene usually induces ovulation (anti-oestrogen, and blocks the inhibition of FSH) and is tried before gonadotrophins or wedge resection of the ovaries.

If fertility is not required the Combined Pill is advised, because ovulation occasionally occurs and also the progesterone protects against carcinoma caused by the high oestrogen levels.

Fat is thought to initiate or aggravate the condition, therefore weight loss should be advised.

Hirsutism

Hirsutism is a common complaint and causes a lot of anxiety about both appearance and loss of femininity.

Males and females have the same number of hair follicles at birth. Hirsutism is due to sensitization of male pattern hair follicles by testosterone, possibly due to a temporary fall in sex hormone binding globulin (SHBG) and a rise in free testosterone levels. Once activated, the hair continues to grow (hence hair tends to recur on stopping drug treatment).

A full history and examination is important. Ask about drugs (e.g. Phenytoin, minoxidil, danazol or combined pills containing norgestrel), periods and family history. Examine to see full extent of hirsutism and to exclude signs of virilization (breast atrophy, cliteromegaly, unusual musculature). If hirsutism is mild and periods regular the woman can be reassured.

The following would indicate referral to a gynaecological endocrinologist, to exclude virilizing tumours (which can be life-threatening):

— Rapid progression of hair growth
— Reduced menses or infertility
— Virilization
— Hair on the shoulders
— Late onset acne

Constitutional hirsutism

98% of cases are constitutional. The hirsutism is usually confined to the face and forearms and starts to develop from the time of puberty. This is usually a family history and it is particularly common in Southern European women. Periods are regular. Serum testosterone (a useful single screening test) is normal and can be a useful way of reassuring about femininity. Low SHBG levels usually predicts a good response to oestrogens.

Treatment is systemic or cosmetic.

Systemic treatment

— Dexamethasone 0.5 mg daily (suppression of androgens)
— Oestrogens (to elevate SHBG levels)
— Cyproterone acetate (anti-androgen)
— Spironolactone (anti-androgen)

First-line treatment is a combined pill, e.g. Minovlar (ethinyloestradiol 50 g, Norethisterone 1 mg) which helps in 50%. The drug Diane (ethinyloestradiol 50 g, cyproterone acetate 2 mg) is particularly useful if there is also acne. More severe cases of hirsutism may respond to higher doses of cyproterone, 50 mg–100 mg daily, combined with 50 g ethinyloestradiol for menstrual regulation and contraception (cyproterone can feminize a male fetus). Lethargy and breast tenderness sometimes occur but are usually mild. The initial course of treatment is 18–24 months. Improvement takes 3–6 months (the growth cycle of the hair follicle).

Topical therapy   Important because systemic therapy is longterm and hirsutism recurs when it is stopped. The mainstay of therapy is epilation. None of the depilatory methods increase hair growth. Methods include:

— shaving
— electrolysis
— waxing
— depilatory creams
— plucking
— depilatory gloves
— bleaching
— cosmetic make-up

Raised androgen levels   Rarely, hirsutism is due to raised androgen levels. Periods become scanty. The possibilities are:

a) polycystic ovary syndrome (POS)
b) virilizing tumours (adrenal, ovary)
c) CAH
d) Cushing's syndrome

   a) POS is suspected from the associated obesity and oligo-menorrhoea. Laparoscopy may show the typical polycystic ovaries. The hirsutism may respond to the pill or can be treated with cyproterone acetate (an anti-androgen) but this is highly teratogenic and the woman must also be on the pill. It takes 6–12 months to work (the growth cycle of the hair follicle).

   b) Virilizing tumours are suspected if hirsutism is pre-pubertal or suddenly develops some years after puberty or if there are other signs of virilization, particularly clitoral hypertrophy (and later deep voice, muscular development, breast atrophy, bitemporal balding and acne). Serum testosterone levels are very high. Laparotomy and splitting the ovaries may be necessary to look for a small hilar cell tumour or adrenal scans and catheterization of the adrenal veins.

   c) Mild CAH can present late and is diagnosed by raised urinary 17 oxo-steroids and raised plasma 17-hydroxy-progesterone (or its urinary metabolite prengnanetriol). Cortisone replacement cures the problem.

   d) Cushing's syndrome is suspected from obesity, striae, glycosuria and hypertension. Diagnosis is confirmed by raised midnight cortisol and failure to suppress cortisol with low dose dexamethasone (or, best of all, a raised 24-hour urinary free cortisol). The cause is distinguished by:

1. High-dose dexamethasone test (a pituitary tumour will be suppressed)
2. ACTH assay (high if ectopic, e.g. oat cell carcinoma, low if adrenal tumour)
3. Urinary 17 oxo-steroids (high if adrenal carcinoma, low if adenoma)

Infertility   The problem of infertility can largely be managed by the interested GP. About 10% of couples are involuntarily infertile. 1 in 6 of the population require help at some time in their lives because of infertility. 1 in 8 need help to have a first child and many will fail. The average time for the normal couple to conceive is 6 cycles. 90% of *fertile couples* achieve pregnancy by 1 year and investigation is normally delayed until after 1 year of regular intercourse (at least twice a week). The causes are:

— coital factors
— defective ovulation (30%)
— defective sperm (30%)
— tubal blockage (20%)
— endometriosis (6%)
— hostile cervical mucus (5%)

The investigations may take 6–24 months and usually all of them are done because two or three sub-optimal features may be present. If the prognosis is hopeless the couple should be told and AID or adoption may be considered. In 20% all the tests appear normal and no cause is found, but anxiety may be a factor because couples sometimes achieve pregnancy while under investigation.

Often the woman presents first, but the woman and her partner should be seen together whenever possible. It takes two to be infertile and male factors are involved in at least a third of cases.

A possible scheme of management is as follows:

1. Detailed history and examination of both partners. The problem should be taken seriously at the initial presentation. The couple will normally be hoping for referral and delay in referral can be misconstrued as lack of interest. It is usually best to counsel about the optimum timing for intercourse (and pre-ovulation mucus charges) and to refer early to a specialist clinic (not all consultants are interested in infertility). Ongoing advice, explanation and support are especially important for couples as they face a series of investigations and often long periods of waiting for the results of tests. For the 50% who fail to conceive the support of an interested GP is particularly important.

The GP should:

— take a smear
— screen for rubella antibodies
— check chlamydial antibody titres
— arrange seminal analysis

If chlamydial antibodies are high there is a high chance of tubal damage needing early investigation. Seminal analysis needs to be interpreted with caution unless there is obvious severe oligospermia.

2. It is always safe to treat with clomiphene 100 mg daily on days 2–6 of each cycle. If this is unsuccessful, or if there is oligomenorrhoea, check:

— Prolactin (hyperprolactinaemia)
— T4, TSH (hypothyroidism)
— FSH (premature menopause)
— Progesterone assay day 20–25 of cycle.

3. If pregnancy has not been achieved on clomiphene await specialist appointment. Send detailed letter plus all results. The following tests may be needed:

— post-coital tests
— progesterone assays
— repeat hormone assays
— skull x-rays
— laparoscopy
— dilation and curretage
— tubal insufflation

Liaise with specialists and maintain contact with couple for explanation and support. It is better to use the word 'subfertile' while the couple are still undergoing tests.

4. Postcoital test. If poor, repeat history, examination and seminal analysis. If non-motile and the smear showed chlamydia, repeat the test after a course of tetracycline; otherwise give mid-cycle oestrogens (ethinyloestrodiol 20 μg Days 11, 12, 13 and 14), to improve the quality of cervical mucus, and repeat the test. If still non-motile; arrange:

— sperm mucus penetration tests (in vitro)
— anti-sperm antibody measurement (male and female)

5. If cycles are anovular and clomiphene is unsuccessful then ovulation is induced with human menopausal gonadotrophin and HCG or LHRH. Peak progesterone values under 35 nmol/l despite stimulation is designated 'inadequate luteal phase'.

6. The commonest class of infertility is unexplained. Up to three years the chances of conceiving are good. After 3 years the chances diminish dramatically but IVF can still be successful in many of these couples. Measurement of pregnancy specific glycoprotein suggests menstrual abortion accounts for a proportion of these cases

N.B. Temperature charting is usually unnecessary with the advent of progesterone assays and increases anxiety without aiding management.

Notes   1. The couple should be seen together initially so they both clearly understand what will be involved. Ask about intercourse (technique and frequency) remembering that 'infertility' may be their way of presenting a psychosexual problem (vaginismus or impotence).

Ask the woman about her cycle (regularity, pain) dyspareunia, infections (post-partum or post-abortion) and gonorrhoea, and examine for fibroids or tenderness (endometriosis, infection).

Ask the man about his job (prolonged sitting can increase testicular temperature — e.g. driving) his general health (diet, exercise, smoking, alcohol), recent high fevers, drugs, previous infections and operations. Bilateral mumps orchitis or late orchidopexy for undescended testes can cause oligospermia. Gonorrhoea or hernioraphy can damage and obstruct the vas deferens. TUR can cause retrograde ejaculation.

Examine standing for a varicocele, exclude hypospadias, assess testicular size, palpate the vas for thickening and perform a PR for tenderness (prostatitis).

N.B. A hydrocele does not affect fertility.

2. Both the basal temperature charts and a special thermo-meter with $0.1°C$ readings can be prescribed. Explain that the oral temperature must be taken before rising every morning. Ovulation can occur 3 days either side of the rise in temperature. Temperature charting has been largely superseded by assay of serum progesterone, measured on Day 21 (when it should be above 30 nmol/l). If this is low, it confirms anovulation and treatment with clomiphene (Clomid) is indicated. Clomiphene is an anti-oestrogen that prevents oestrogen from inhibiting FSH — the FSH rise then initiates a normal cycle and ovulation.

Give clomiphene 50 mg daily for Days 1–5 of the cycle and continue the charts. If unsuccessful, try 100 mg Days 1–5 then 200 mg Days 1–5. If this is unsuccessful, exclude hyperpro-lactaemia or hypothyroidism. If the woman has amenorrhoea, a progesterone bleed will show that it is due to anovular cycles that will respond to clomiphene.

If clomiphene is unsuccessful, then Pergonal (FSH acquired from postmenopausal urine) has to be used, at a special centre. Urinary oestrogens are monitored to prevent over-stimulation (causing ovarian cysts and multiple births). An injection of HCG (LH-like action) is given to stimulate ovulation, and the best time for this can be predicted by ultrasound scan (showing the ripe follicle bulging).

Serial scans throughout the cycle may reveal explanations for infertility (luteinized unruptured follicle syndrome, poor follicle development, persistence of cysts) and should be combined with serial measurements of oestrogens, progesterones and gonadoptrophic hormones. Simple rapid radioimmuno-assays are now available for measuring progesterone in saliva and in capillary blood collected on filter paper after finger prick. These techniques allow daily specimens to be collected at home for subsequent assessment at the end of the cycle.

3. The postcoital test is the single most useful test in infertility. Cervical mucus is taken around Day 14 of the cycle, the morning after intercourse, and should show at least 10 motile sperms per HPF. Accurate timing is essential and the test needs special

experience to interpret properly. If the count is normal it proves that:

— coitus is effective
— cervical mucus is adequate (implying ovulation)
— sperm is normal

Sperm penetration of pre-ovulatory cervical mucus is twice as good as seminal analysis at predicting fertility.

If the test is poor and seminal analysis is normal, sperm mucus penetration tests may show sperm clumping and poor penetration (look for anti-sperm antibodies in the man's serum) or sperm immobilization by mucus (look for antibodies in the woman's serum). Intracervical insemination of fresh semen at the time of ovulation can be tried.

4. The best test for tubal patency is laparoscopy and hydro-tubation with methylene blue. The success rate of tubal surgery is low (20%), whether

— salpingolysis (for adhesions)
— salpingostomy (for fimbrial blockage)
— re-implantation (for cornual blockage)

The alternative is *in vitro* fertilization, which involves LH measurements, laparoscopic collection of the ovum in follicular fluid at the time of the LH surge, incubation with sperm and re-injection through the cervix at about the 16-cell stage. Success is also about 20%.

5. Endometriosis probably interferes with ovum release. Excision of chocolate cysts can restore fertility. Treatment with danazol restores fertility in about 50%.

Male infertility If the sperm count is poor, seminal analysis should always be repeated because there is daily fluctuation, and fevers (e.g. influenza) can cause a low count for 3 months. A masturbation specimen collected after 2–3 days abstinence in a sterile plastic container should be examined by an experienced seminologist within 2 hours.

There should be at least:

— 2 ml
— 20 million/ml
— 75% motile
— 75% normal morphology

A *low count* may be due to:

— drugs (sulphasalazine, cyclophosphamide, nitrofurantoin)
— varicocele (examine standing)
— raised testicular temperature
— prostatitis
— testicular atrophy (trauma, infection, hypopituitarism, XXY)

In unexplained infertility where seminal analysis is normal more refined tests may be indicated e.g. zona-free hamster egg penetration test or more refined tests of sperm motility e.g. timed exposure photomicrography, videomicrography or laser Doppler velocimetry.

Management

1. Consider drugs or excessive alcohol. If a varicocele is present, bilateral supra-inguinal ligation of the spermatic veins can restore fertility in 70%. If the testes are small and there is gynaecomastia, exclude Kleinfelter's syndrome (XXY) by chromosomal analysis.

2. Otherwise advise cold scrotal douches, avoiding hot baths, boxer shorts, regular exercise and stopping smoking, and repeat the seminal analysis in 3 months (each wave of sperm takes 3 months to develop).

3. If prostatitis is suspected (tenderness PR) a 3-month course of rotating antibiotics (e.g. septrin, erythromycin, tetracycline) can sometimes improve the count.

4. If the count remains low then tamoxifen or clomiphene (to increase FSH), or mesterolone 100 mg daily for a year, can be tried. (Testosterone inhibits FSH and actually lowers the count). There is no evidence that these empirical treatments help.

5. Finally, vitamin B or arginine have their advocates. It is reasonable to try short courses of empirical treatment when no other treatment has been effective. Remember that even very low counts are not a complete bar to fertility, and it is best to maintain some hope (which also causes less disharmony if the woman achieves pregnancy by extramarital means).

6. Note that hormone assays and testicular biopsy are not routinely necessary. Pituitary failure will be suspected clinically (tiredness, impotence, pale hairless skin). Degeneration of the seminiferous tubules may be suspected from small testes but biopsy does not alter management.

7. If there is total aspermia, then FSH and testicular biopsy become useful tests to distinguish blocked ducts (normal testes, normal FSH) from testicular failure (small testes, high FSH, irreversible).

In obstruction, a vasogram can be performed to exclude non-surgical obstruction deep at the ejaculatory ducts and epididy-movasostomy performed (but results are still poor). If no block is demonstrated, testicular biopsy may show spermatogenic arrest (normal FSH) which may respond to Pergonal.

N.B. FSH stimulates sperm production, LH stimulates testosterone secretion.

8. If the sperm count is normal, the man may still be responsible due to serum IgG anti-sperm antibodies (suspected by clumping of sperm on a postcoital test). It is difficult to treat, but giving him a course of steroids the week before the woman's period can be tried.

9. Infertility due to cervical hostility, hypospadias or poor sperm volume may be overcome by AIH.

In vitro fertilization (IVF)   In vitro fertilization was first reported in 1959 in rabbits. Edwards and Steptoe reported fertilization of human oocytes in vitro in 1970 and successful re-implantation in 1976. The first 'test-tube' baby was born in 1978. In 1981 it was demonstrated that IVF and successful embryo transfer (ET) could be achieved in controlled cycles as well as natural cycles, making the prediction of ovulation time more accurate. In 1983 embryos were successfully frozen and implanted, allowing repeated attempts at ET without the need for repeated attempts at oocyte recovery.

The *pregnancy rate* varies from 10–20% depending on the number of embryos transferred. If one embryo is replaced the chances of pregnancy are about 10%, replacing two increases this to 15%, three to 20% and four to 25%. More than four increases the risks of multiple pregnancy or miscarriage. (A 25% pregnancy rate approaches that for the pregnancy rate per natural cycle in a sexually active woman of 25 who is not using contraception.) The chances of having an abnormal baby are probably no different to natural conception.

Indications for IVF   The technique was initially used for patients with irreparable tube damage, but since then it has been successful for other types of infertility:

— tubal occlusion, distortion or ablation
— pelvic endometriosis
— sperm problems (oligospermia, antibodies, cervical hostility)
— ovulatory problems (e.g. polycytic ovaries with no oocyte release)
— unexplained infertility

Referral for IVF   The first step is referral to an IVF unit where the team includes doctors, nurses, theatre staff, embryologist, laboratory technicians and ultrasound personnel. The couple are seen together and counselled about the procedure. A full history and examination of both partners and semen analysis precede a laparoscopy to assess the access to the ovaries and length of uterine cavity and to dilate the cervix prior to embryo transfer. IVF treatment can be undertaken on a day-care basis and is usually organised by the IVF *programme co-ordinator*. The treatment involves two weeks of serial scans and blood tests, HCG injection around Day 12, egg collection 36 hours later (by laparoscope or by aspiration under ultrasound control) and then embryo transfer two days later, performed in the lithotomy position without sedation. The woman then waits to see if the next period is missed.

NOTE: There are now 25 centres in Britain carrying out

IVF, only one operated by the NHS. The waiting list is around 2–4 years and the cost is £1,000–£2,500 per treatment.

The procedure involves:

1. *Follicle stimulation.* Drugs are usually used to induce multiple follicle development rather than relying on the natural cycle because the success rate rises if several embryos are transferred at once. This means there is an increased risk of multiple births (about 15% of pregnancies). The drugs used are Clomiphine (Clomid), human menopausal gonadotrophin (Pergonal), Tamoxifen (Nolvadex) or pure FSH (Metrodin).

2. *Serial scans* are performed to monitor follicle growth and endometrial response (which correlates closely with good follicle development) and serial plasma oestradiol measurements are taken. The diameter of the pre-ovulatory follicle varies from 11–24 mm, so scan alone cannot predict ovulation. The scan shows the number and site of developing follicles and excludes recent ovulation.

3. *HCG injection* to stimulate ovulation (which allows oocyte collection 36 hours later). The timing of HCG administration is vital and should be given when follicular development is complete and just before the endogenous surge of LH. If the LH surge has occurred ovulation will be sooner than expected. LH levels are therefore measured at this time.

4. *Oocyte recovery* by laparoscopy or aspiration of pre-ovulatory follicles under ultrasound control. The ultrasound method of aspiration can be painful but has advantages when the ovaries are inaccessible to the laparoscope — e.g. following surgery or inflammation. The aspiration needle route may be percutaneous, then transvesical (i.e. through the bladder), urethral or vaginal. This can be run as a day-care service.

5. A *Sperm specimen* is collected and prepared in culture medium.

6. *Fertilization.* The oocytes are washed in culture media and allowed to incubate for six hours before mixing with sperm. Fertilization is recognized by the presence of pronuclei 12–16 hours later. The technique of incubating the oocytes prior to insemination has increased the success rate (failure of fertilization occurs in 10%).

7. *Embryo transfer.* The patient returns 36 hours later for embryo transfer (no sedation is needed). The embryo is transferred transcervically and implantation can be successful at any stage from pro-nuclei development to blastocyst. There is no evidence that hormone therapy in the luteal phase increases the success rate.

IVF — The possibilities

Sperm donation (AID) is available if there is an associated male infertility factor. *Ovum donation* can be used to achieve pregnancy in patients with premature menopause or ovarian dysgenesis, provided hormonal support is administered. Many women undergoing sterilization are willing to donate eggs.

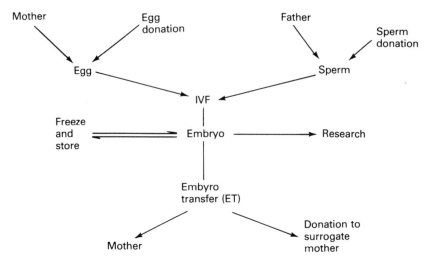

Fig. 1

Cryopreservation of embryos was reported in 1983 and it allows storage of spare embryos for repeated attempts at embryo transfer without the need for repeated attempts at oocyte recovery. Only about 1 in 10 embryos transferred survives in the womb, and freezing of embryos allows repeated attempts to be made.

Surrogate motherhood ('womb-leasing'), whether by ET or by insemination, is deemed illegal.

The ethical issues of IVF

The Warnock Report (1984) was the government's answer to public concern over the social, ethical and legal issues of IVF in terms of both the treatment of infertility and research on human embryos.

The main recommendations were:

1. A new statutory *licensing authority* to regulate both infertility services and research projects.

2. IVF clinics (and AID clinics) should be *licensed*.

3. Services for IVF should be expanded within the NHS.

4. Agencies (commercial or otherwise) recruiting women for *surrogate pregnancies* ('womb-leasing') should be illegal (but individuals entering into private surrogacy arrangements will not be liable to criminal prosecution).

5. *Children* born by IVF or AID should not be branded as illegitimate (and changes in legislation were recommended).

6. *Egg donation* should be accepted and subject to the same controls as AID.

7. *Embryo donation* should be accepted provided that the semen and egg are brought together in vitro.

8. *Spare embryos* may be frozen and stored for repeated

attempts. The right to use or dispose of the embryos should pass to the storage authority after ten years (or in the event of the death of both parents).

9. *Research* on embryos should be legal up to fourteen days, (when the primitive streak appears), and it should be legal to create embryos solely for experimentation (e.g. rescuing ova from women undergoing sterilization and fertilizing them from a donor bank).

Embryo research Some people are opposed to embryo research, taking the view that a human being is created at the moment of fertilization. Most people accept that an embryo does not command the rights and privileges of a fully formed person, and that research on human embryos will bring important advances for the benefit of the community. Allowing research up to *fourteen days* is a compromise between these two views, although many feel that six weeks would be more realistic.

Embryo research may yield important new information on cell interaction, *cell differentiation*, tissue organisation and the causation of congenital malformations and methods of prevention. It may become possible to diagnose *genetic disorders* in the blastocyst prior to implantation (avoiding the need for late termination) and techniques of *gene insertion* may one day cure diseases due to defective genes.

Current research is concentrating on ways of *improving IVF*. Individual centres are researching on a new contraceptive pill, male infertility and genetic abnormalities in the pre-embryo (the term for the fertilised ovum up to day fourteen).

Habitual abortion This is defined as three or more consecutive miscarriages. The causes are:

— cervical incompetence (mid-trimester)
— abnormal uterine cavity (mid-trimester)
— chromosomal abnormality
— systemic illness (exclude SLE)
— unknown (50%)

1. Try to confirm that previous episodes of amenorrhoea followed by bleeding were abortions and not simply dysfunctional bleeding. Ask about:

— pattern of amenorrhoea and bleeds
— was the fetus seen?
— were villi seen on curettings? (old notes)

2. Painless mid-trimester abortions suggest cervical incompetence. There will be a history of terminations or cervical surgery. Diagnosed, in between pregnancies, by a hysterosalpingogram demonstrating that the whole cervical canal is wider than 10 mm. Treatment is by cervical encirclage suture inserted at 16 weeks (after any potential abortion due to fetal abnormality)

and removed at 36 weeks (before spontaneous labour might start).

3. Congenital abnormalities of the uterus or submucus fibroids can be excluded by a hysterosalpingogram. Abnormalities such as bicornuate or septate uterus can be corrected surgically.

4. Chromosomal abnormalities (e.g. balanced translocations) in either parent can cause recurrent abortions and chromosomal analysis should be performed on both parents and the fetus if aborted.

5. Maternal illness. Ask about high fevers in previous pregnancies which could account for abortion. Enquire about general health and exclude particularly diabetes, syphilis, SLE, hypothyroidism and haemoglobinopathies.

6. These patients are always anxious. Scans are useful to confirm pregnancy and monitor growth. Forbid coitus. Bedrest is usually recommended. Progesterone therapy is only helpful in early (e.g. 6 weeks) abortions due to a corpus luteal defect, when hydroxy-progesterone 250 mg i.m. is given twice weekly from the time of diagnosis to 20 weeks. Folate can be a useful placebo treatment but there is no evidence that it is effective.

Threatened abortion

About 10–15% of all pregnancies end as a miscarriage, almost always due to fetal abnormality. Many occur very early and get diagnosed as 'heavy periods'. The rest usually occur around 10–12 weeks.

Painless vaginal bleeding in early pregnancy is diagnosed as *threatened abortion*. (Rarely it can be due to a painless ectopic). Three out of four cases settle down, when there is no increased risk of fetal abnormality, although it would be regarded as an 'at risk' pregnancy.

Ask whether pregnancy has been confirmed by urine tests or scan, and if not, consider that it may be simply dysfunctional bleeding. There is no evidence that any form of treatment helps but the usual advice is bedrest until it stops and avoid coitus for 2 weeks. 50 μg of Anti-D should be given if the woman is Rhesus negative. When bleeding has settled, pass a speculum to exclude a cervical polyp and take a smear. An ultrasound scan should be arranged to confirm the presence of a fetal heart.

An abortion becomes *inevitable* if there is:

— fetal death
— heavy bleeding
— low abdominal pain
— cervical dilatation
— products of conception are passed

VE to assess the cervix. Removing any products trapped in the cervix often decreases bleeding and shock. If the bleeding is heavy, give 0.5 mg ergometrine (i.v. or i.m.). If there is heavy bleeding — usually mid-trimester — call a flying squad to transfuse the patient. Otherwise, admit for curettage, because in most cases abortion will be incomplete and haemorrhage or infection can develop. Afterwards the Hb is checked and broad spectrum antibiotics given if fever or discharge develop. The woman is sometimes advised to use contraception for 3 months (to allow a normal endometrium to regenerate).

If the woman is seen a day or so after an abortion, signs that it is *incomplete* are:

— continual bleeding
— cervix still open
— bulky, tender uterus

Curettage will be necessary. Some specialists advocate curettage after every abortion, even seemingly complete abortions, to prevent later haemorrhage or infection.

Tubal pregnancy 1 in 500 pregnancies in this country are ectopic and almost all of these are tubal. Usually the cause is unknown but there may be a history of:

— tubal surgery (infertility or sterilization)
— IUCD or POP
— pelvic sepsis
— gonorrhoea
— (tuberculosis)

The Fallopian tube gets gradually wider (cornua, isthmus, ampulla, infundibulum) and there are two clinical pictures depending on which part of the tube is affected. Both are characterized by a history of:

— a missed period
— dizziness or fainting
— abdominal pain that PRECEDES:
— slight vaginal bleeding.

1. *90% are ampullary*, occuring in the free end of the fallopian tube, and rupture or abortion occurs at 6–9 weeks gestation. Abdominal pain can be colicky (tubal peristalsis) or continuous, sometimes with shoulder-tip pain (due to bleeding from the tube).

Vaginal bleeding can be slight and dark (prune juice), coming from the endometrial decidua no longer supported by HCG, or it can be fresh red bleeding coming down from the tube.

VE shows marked tenderness on moving the cervix. The uterus may feel bulky, and sometimes a tender pulsatile mass is felt in one fornix or a large posterior mass (pelvic haematoma).

Differential diagnosis is from:

— threatened abortion (bleeding then pain)
— salpingitis (fever, bilateral tenderness)
— appendicitis (fever, furred tongue, nausea, diarrhoea)
— ovarian cyst: torsion or rupture (no bleeding)

An ultrasound showing a definite gestation sac in the uterus excludes the diagnosis. *If an ectopic is suspected, laparoscopy is performed* and if free blood is seen in the peritoneum, laparotomy and salpingectomy.

N.B. Diagnosis is notoriously difficult, and tubal pregnancy can be painless and present merely as a late 'period'. If tubal pregnancy is suspected a laparoscopy is indicated.

2. *10% occur in the interstitial part* of the tube (isthmus or cornua) and tend to rupture early and externally with massive intraperitoneal haemorrhage. The woman's period may only be late by a few days when she develops severe abdominal pain, shock, and generalized abdominal tenderness and rebound (with slight distension). There may be no vaginal bleeding. The important point is to *operate immediately* and resuscitate simultaneously. VE should be avoided as it does not contribute to the diagnosis and may make the haemorrhage worse.

Pruritis vulvae
— vaginal discharge
— glycosuria,
— incontinence.
— infection (candida, warts)
— infestation (threadworms, scabies, lice)
— skin disorder (eczema, psoriasis, generalized pruritus)
— contact sensitivity
— vulval dystrophy
— psychogenic

Diagnosis can be difficult because scratching causes secondary hypertrophic changes. Ask about vaginal discharge, inspect carefully, swab if necessary and remember threadworms (especially in children). Always exclude glycosuria.

Treat any infection, remembering to treat the partner if necessary. Stop all applications. Contact sensitivity (to deodorants, spermicides, antiseptics) can be proved by patch testing. If vulval dystrophy is suspected, refer for biopsy.

If no cause is found, treat with a 1–2 week course of a mild topical steroid (e.g. 1% hydrocortisone) and an oral antihistamine at night e.g. promethazine (Phenergan) 50 mg, which is also a sedative and has a 12-hour action.

Recommend regular washing (perineal micro-organisms contaminate the vulva, particularly in the elderly), careful drying (a hair dryer is useful) and avoidance of tight nylon underwear or nightwear (warmth and moisture cause maceration)

Pruritus vulvae is not infrequently a symptom which may point to underlying psychological problems, which may be of a psychosexual nature.

Vulval dystrophy
1. Primary atrophy (thin skin — red and shiny)
2. Lichen sclerosis (thick skin — white plaques)

Chronic vulvitis of any cause can progress to dystrophy.

Primary atrophy is premenopausal and does not respond to oestrogens. It must be followed up, because dysplastic white patches can develop.

Lichen sclerosis resembles localized scleroderma and usually extends to the perianal region.

Both cause intense itching and both are premalignant. If suspected, and particularly if a fissure develops, biopsies of the area must be taken. If histology shows dysplasia (loss of differentiation of squamous cells) or intra-epithelial carcinoma, it is treated with topical 5-fluorouracil or by simple vulvectomy. If left, 20% progress over about 10 years to invasive carcinoma.

Vulval carcinoma is treated by radical vulvectomy (total vulvectomy plus inguinal lymphadenectomy) and the overall 5YS is 50%.

Vaginal discharge   Vaginal secretions are normally acidic and protective. Oestrogens increase the glycogen content of vaginal squames and the commensal lactobacilli metabolize the glycogen to acid. This protective acidity is decreased before puberty, after the menopause, with broad-spectrum antibiotics and with vaginal douches or excessive cervical discharge (which is alkaline), which all predispose to infection.

Vaginal discharge is a common complaint. In 80% of cases a pathological discharge is due to candidiasis or trichomoniasis. Clinically there are three situations.

1. Physiological
2. Specific infection (trichomoniasis, candidiasis, gonorrhoea, *H. vaginalis*)
3. Mucopurulent or blood-stained

The diagnosis is usually obvious from the history:

— colour, smell, itchiness, soreness
— sudden (infection)
— symptoms in the partner
— pill, antibiotics, steroids (*Candida*)
— douches, pessaries (sensitivity)
— recent delivery or abortion

Increased physiological discharge (leucorrhoea) causes no odour or itch, though it may stain slightly. Unlike other causes, it contains no pus cells. It can increase due to:

— vaginal transudate (sexual excitement)
— cervical erosion (pill, pregnancy)
— ovulatory cascade of cervical mucus
— tail of IUCD

If there is pus or blood, consider:

— vaginitis (atrophic, foreign body tampon or ring pessary)

— cervicitis
— salpingitis
— endometritis (i.e., puerperal sepsis)
— carcinoma or polyp

Management

1. Examine the abdomen for tenderness (salpingitis)
2. Note any vulvitis. Pass a speculum, inspect the cervix and take a smear. If gonorrhoea is suspected, try to milk pus from the urethra and take charcoal swabs from urethra and cervix into Stuart's medium. Otherwise take an ordinary HVS.
3. Perform a bimanual examination.
4. Chronic cervicitis is treated by cryocautery. Any persistent unexplained discharge is an indication for curettage.
5. In a postmenopausal woman, a bloodstained discharge is an indication for curettage to exclude endometrial carcinoma — even if there is atrophic vaginitis.
6. In a child, the combination of an under-oestrogenized vagina and poor hygiene may cause a bacterial infection. PR may reveal a foreign body and EUA, using a nasal speculum, may be needed to remove it.

Candidiasis (thrush)

Candida albicans is a gut commensal and should not be present in the vagina. Predisposing factors to vaginal candidiasis are:

— the pill
— pregnancy
— broad-spectrum antibiotics
— steroids
— diabetes

The clinical features are itching, soreness, dyspareunia, redness and a thick white discharge with white curds. On VE grey irremovable patches may be seen on erythematous areas. It can be symptomless. Treatment is with antifungal pessaries and cream (e.g. nystatin, clotrimazole or miconazole). Recurrent thrush is common, often due to a combination of the pill and tight nylon underwear.

Management of recurrent thrush involves

— exclude diabetes
— treat the partner (the balantitis can be symptomless)
— prophylaxis if antibiotics are prescribed with the pill
— regular prophylaxis (e.g. pessaries mid-cycle)
— systemic therapy with ketoconazole (Nizoral) 200 mg daily — not in pregnancy or with liver disease. There is a 1 in 10,000 chance of drug-induced hepatitis.

Trichomoniasis

Trichomonas vaginalis is a flagellate protozoan that is acquired venereally. It can cause a profuse frothy green discharge, pruritis, soreness, dyspareunia (sometimes dysuria) and intense inflammation. However, like thrush, it can be completely symptomless. It can be diagnosed by:

— swab and culture
— cervical smear (the protozoa also get stained)
— microscopy of a drop of discharge in saline (the organisms resemble the leucocytes but are motile)

Treatment is with metronidazole (Flagyl) 200 mg t.d.s. for 7 days and the partner must be treated simultaneously. Alcohol must be avoided during treatment (headache, flushing, vomiting, hypotension). An alternative is nimorazole (Naxogin 500).

The cervix

1. The squamo-columnar junction can become everted due to differential growth stimulated by oestrogens (puberty, pregnancy and the pill). The columnar epithelium becomes visible, causing the common but wrongly-named erosion. 50% of women on the pill have an erosion, but treatment by cryo-cautery is only necessary if it is causing a symptomatic discharge.

2. The exposed columnar epithelium undergoes metaplasia to squamous epithelium and the S–C junction moves back into the canal. Nabothian cysts, which resemble tiny sebaceous cysts, can occur where this squamous metaplasia has blocked underlying mucosal crypts causing retention cysts.

3. These Nabothian cysts can become secondarily infected with mixed organisms — chronic cervicitis, causing discharge, dyspareunia and sometimes pain. Antibiotics are usually in-effective and treatment is by cryocautery in outpatients, which takes about 10 minutes. It may cause a watery discharge for 2–3 weeks.

4. A cervical polyp causes non-menstrual bleeding. If the pedicle is visible it can be twisted off, but should be sent for histology.

Cervical smears

1. The screening programme is based on the assumption that carcinoma-in-situ progresses to invasive carcinoma of the cervix. There are many recorded cases of this happening (no longer ethical) and premalignant changes are usually seen surrounding an invasive carcinoma, implying that the one develops into the other. The peak incidence of carcinoma-in-situ (35 years) and carcinoma (45 years) suggests about a 10-year natural history (still not proved).

However, the incidence of precancer is about twice that of cancer suggesting that about half of the cases with dysplasia return to normal and never become invasive.

Among screened women, the treatment of pre-invasive carcinoma has undoubtedly reduced the incidence of invasive carcinoma. Unfortunately the women most at risk tend to use the service the least.

2. Routine smears should be done every three years in all sexually-active women. Always inspect the cervix, because a necrotic tumour can give a negative result. About 1 in 10 cases of carcinoma-in-situ are missed (false negatives) but by repeating the first smear at one year this is reduced to 1 in 100.

3. A smear is taken from the squamo-columnar junction, the active region where carcinoma first develops. None of the conditions giving rise to abnormal smears can be seen with naked eye inspection. It is important to sample the SCJ all round the os because only one small focus may be involved. A smear gives an estimate of the degree of abnormality in the cervix but it cannot determine the site or size of the lesion. The spatula should be wiped 3 or 4 times along the length of the slide and fixative applied immediately. A smear is easiest to interpret during the follicular phase of the cycle but is useless during a period. Pregnancy, the pill, the IUCD or a polyp will change the appearance of the cells and must be mentioned on the form.

4. *The result*:

1 — inadequate specimen
2 — negative
3 — mild dysplasia
4 — severe dysplasia
5 — ca-in-situ
6 — 7 glandular neoplasia
7 — inflammatory
 — trichomonas
 — candida
 — viral
 — severe

The cytologist looks at the size of nuclei and nuclear/cytoplasmic ratio. Normal cells develop a smaller nucleus as they migrate up from the basal layer. In malignant transformation epithelial turnover increases and causes immature cells with larger nuclei to reach the surface (dyskaryotic cells).

N.B. Dyskaryosis on cytology implies dysplasia will be found on histology. Occasionally the term atypia is used to mean dyskaryosis.

5. *Management*:
Inflammatory (large nucleus but cytoplasm degenerated) treat the cause and repeat smear in 2 months (after epithelium has regenerated). If second smear is inflammatory refer for colposcopy.

Mild dysplasia	— repeated smear and annual smears now indicated.
Mild dysplasia × 2—	colposcopy
Severe dysplasia	— colposcopy
Carcinoma-in-situ	— colposcopy

6. The UK screening service has been a relative failure compared to other countries. Since 1968 it has resulted in only a 13% reduction in mortality compared to 50–60% in some countries.

The death rate in women under 35 has actually risen

(presumably because sexual activity has risen) despite the intensive routine screening in this age group. There has been a dramatic increase in precancerous lesions in women under 35.

Many women over 35 (known to be the group at most risk of progression to invasive disease) are still being missed.

Because of this, a DHSS working party (1981) has recommended that the current policy (screening after the third pregnancy or 5-yearly from 35) be revised. They propose that all sexually-active women should have smears:

— at 22
— in each pregnancy (no recall system needed)
— at 30 (if no smear for the past 5 years)
— 35–65 (all women must be recalled 5-yearly)

They calculated that this would only require the 2.8 million smears per year already being taken, and would significantly reduce the incidence of carcinoma of the cervix. There is now evidence to suggest smears should be advised every 3 years for maximum safety. The presence of human papillomavirus indicates annual smears.

A systematic recall system and age/sex register is fundamental to a screening programme. The link with the wart virus may alter screening policy.

Colposcopy and Ablative Therapy

Until the mid 1970s the standard treatment for cervical intra-epithelial neoplasia (CIN) was cone biopsy. The colposcope was pioneered by Stafl in the United States. In 1982 the RCOG concluded that 'ideally no patient with CIN should be treated unless there has been prior colposcopic assessment'. In conjunction with ablative methods of treatment the colposcope allows patients to be diagnosed and treated in outpatients with few complications.

Colposcopy determines:

— site of lesion
— suitability for local destruction
— whether lesion extends to vagina

Cone biopsy has to be performed on all cases where colposcopy is not available.

The colposcope is a microscope with a powerful light source mounted on a stand. The cervix is exposed with a bi-valve speculum with the patent in lithotomy. The colposcope remains 10–15 cm away from the perineum and the cervix is magnified ×10.

The cervix is wiped with normal saline. Abnormal epithelium may appear a deeper pink than the normal pale pink squamous epithelium. Next the cervix is painted with 5% acetic acid which is a protein coagulant that stains abnormal immature epithelium white (because immature cells have less glycogen and more cytoplasmic protein). The degree of whiteness of the demarcated area and the coarseness of the vascular pattern visible in the underlying strata, either as dots (punctate) or as a network (mosaic) allows an estimate of the degree of CIN present. A punch biopsy is taken and local destruction therapy applied.

The presence of large atypical vessels (corkscrew or right-angles bifurcations) are associated with invasive foci and indicate cone biopsy. In cases where the lesion extends out of sight into the endocervical canal or where the whole SCJ is not visible, cone biopsy is indicated.

The abnormal vascular patterns associated with epithelial change are:

— punctate (large vessel loops near the surface — moderate dysplasia)
— mosaic (linear punctuations — severe dysplasia)
— abnormal branching vessels — (suggests micro-invasion)

The colposcope allows small biopsies to be taken of suspicious areas. 3% acetic acid swab makes the dysplastic areas turn white and easier to identify for biopsy. Colposcopy allows cervical intra-epithelial neoplasia to be safely treated with conservative methods using local ablative techniques.

The results of the biopsy are graded:

CIN 1   — mild dysplasia
CIN 2   — severe dysplasia
CIN 3   — carcinoma-in-situ
micro-invasion — less than 3 mm through basement membrane

(Histological features of dysplasia include large or abnormal nuclei, reduced cytoplasm and loss of cell stratification, maturation and polarization).

Ablative methods of treatment All methods aim for effective destruction of abnormal areas with minimal risk to fertility. They include:

— diathermy (requires a GA)
— cryocautery
— cold coagulation
— laser

There has recently been a report of suspected cell survival after cryocautery. The area treated by laser heals completely after one month and there is appreciably less discomfort and vaginal discharge. Cold coagulation is quicker than laser therapy (which takes about 20 minutes) and probably equally effective.

Micro-invasion indicates a cone biopsy. If the transformation zone cannot be fully identified because it extends into the cervical canal then cone biopsy is also indicated. One advantage of the colposcope is that if the transformation zone extends onto the vagina (about 4% of women) it can be identified and destroyed. Follow up smears are essential, and if they become abnormal further biopsy is indicated. Suspicious areas can be followed up by repeat colposcopy.

Carcinoma-in-situ The natural history is:

a) Squamous metaplasia of the squamo-columnar junction replacing areas of columnar epithelium extending into the vagina (an erosion). This is normal. It probably occurs because the sensitive columnar epithelium cannot survive the vaginal acid pH. The increased cell turnover of squamous metaplasia may pre-dispose to the cell transformation.
b) Mild dysplasia
c) Severe dysplasia
d) Carcinoma-in-situ
e) Micro-invasive carcinoma (less than 3 mm)
f) Overt carcinoma of the cervix

N.B. Probably all cases of severe dysplasia progress to overt carcinoma

There are 4,000 new cases of carcinoma of the cervix each year in England and Wales and 4× as many new cases of CIN. The average time for early CIN to develop into cancer is around 10 years but an aggressive form of the disease has emerged in recent years affecting particularly younger women and this undoubtedly develops much faster.

Cone biopsy. If histology shows invasion then cone biopsy has to be done. Schiller's test (iodine to stain glycogen in the normal epithelium) can be used to define the amount of cervix that must be removed, and decrease the complications of:

— infection and haemorrhage
— cervical incompetence (25%)
— cervical stenosis
— infertility (loss of cervical mucus)

Annual follow-up smears are essential to detect any recurrence (the bed of the cervix is left to re-epithelialize).

If smears remain abnormal then vaginal hysterectomy with removal of a cuff of vagina is usually advisable.

Carcinoma of the cervix On average a GP will see carcinoma of the cervix about once every 5 years. Most women are over 40 but the incidence in younger woman is rising. The cause seems to be related to coitus and early age of coitus and other associations are probably secondary to this. It is extremely rare in virgins and associated with:

— early marriage
— high parity
— low SEC
— promiscuity
— venereal disease

The carcinogenic agent was thought to be Herpesvirus type 2 or sperm DNA but in 1976 an association was noted with wart virus infection. Human papillomavirus DNA has been identified in cervical cancer tissue and types 16 and 18 are firmly associated with the cancer. The epidemiology of wart virus infection makes it a strong candidate as a causal agent, but that it is only an opportunistic infection still remains a possibility.

Micro-invasive carcinoma causes no signs or symptoms. Once invasive, the classical symptom is non-menstrual bleeding:

— postcoital
— intermenstrual
— postmenopausal

Pain, discharge, fistulae and uraemia are all late features. The overall 5-YS is still only 45% because of late presentation. 90% of recurrences will occur within the first year and survival to 5 years means cure. If the cervix has a nodule or ulcer, refer for immediate biopsy.

The tumour is staged clinically (Table 1). This involves:

— EUA and biopsy
— rectal examination (? parametrial involvement)
— cystoscopy (? bladder involvement)

1. The treatment of choice is now *radiotherapy* in special centres. With average resources the results of radiotherapy are better than surgery and the mortality and morbidity (especially damage to the ureters) is lower. Both methods eliminate un-detected pelvic secondaries (20% of stage 1). The tumour spreads initially by local invasion, then to nodes within the pelvis, therefore intracavity radiation (twice in 10 days) is combined with external beam therapy to the whole pelvis (20 daily doses) to irradiate obturator and iliac nodes.

In the Manchester technique for intracavity irradiation a tube is inserted into the uterus and rubber ovoids into the fornices and these are attached to tubes which deliver the caesium 137 — *the afterload technique*, which reduces contamination of the staff. The vagina is packed to keep the tubes in place and their position is checked by X-ray before treatment starts.

N.B. Wertheim's radical hysterectomy (with BSO, vaginal cuff and regional nodes) is still used in early carcinoma in young

Table 1 Stages of carcinoma of the cervix

STAGE	SPREAD	TREATMENT	5YS (%)
1a.	Cervix (micro-invasive)	Local excision	100
1b.	Cervix (overt)	Radiotherapy	80
2.	Upper vagina (a), parametrium (b)	Radiotherapy	60
3.	Lower vagina (a), pelvic walls (b)	Radical radiotherapy	30
4.	Bladder, rectum or metastases	Palliation	10

women to avoid vaginal stenosis, and if the cancer is very early, an ovary can be conserved. Surgery is the treatment of choice for adenocarcinoma (95% are squamous, 5% are adeno). Surgery is also necessary if intracavity radiation is contra-indicated by:

— History of pelvic infections
— History of pelvic surgery
— Fibroids (necrosis and acute pain)

Pelvic infections can be re-activated; previous surgery may have caused adhesions which pull loops of gut into the pelvis where they will undergo radiation necrosis.

2. Stage 3 is treated by radical radiotherapy to the whole pelvis. High voltage techniques using multiple ports of entry have reduced complications, especially skin burns, but these still occur:

— vaginal stenosis (preventable by regular intercourse)
— haematuria (bladder telangiectasia)
— cystitis
— vesico-vaginal fistula (6 months later)
— ureteric fibrosis and obstruction
— colitis (months or years later)
— adhesions

3. Stage 4 is treated by palliative radiotherapy (pain, leg oedema) and palliative surgery if fistulae have occurred: colostomy, uretero-ileostomy or removal of the tumour bulk with the bladder and rectum (exenteration). The terminal problems are:

— pain
— bleeding, infection (vaginal erosion)
— fistulae
— gut obstruction
— ureteric obstruction

Death is due to renal failure (50%) anaemia, infection or cachexia.

Acute salpingitis

— Puerperal or post-abortal ($\mp$ anaerobes)
— IUCD
— Gonococcal
— Chlamydial

It is due to ascending infection and therefore never seen in pregnancy after 12 weeks when the decidual membranes seal off the tubes. It is always bilateral. The clinical features are:

— bilateral pain and tenderness, dyspareunia
— fever, vomiting
— discharge
— marked tenderness (on moving the cervix and in the fornices)
— urinary symptoms, proctitis.

Urethral and cervical swabs should always be taken to exclude gonorrhoea. HVS is often negative however, and swabs taken at laparoscopy (for both aerobic and anaerobic culture) are needed for definitive diagnosis. Some advocate laparoscopy for all cases to exclude appendicitis, endometriosis, ectopic pregnancy, ovarian tumours and corpus luteal bleeds. In one study 814 cases of PID diagnosed by experienced gynaecologists were laparoscoped and the diagnosis was confirmed in only 532. Laparoscopy is indicated if the diagnosis is in doubt, if the woman is acutely ill, if there is no response to antibiotics and in older women when malignancy is more likely. Prompt treatment with high doses of broad-spectrum antibiotics (e.g. co-trimoxazole, erythromycin and metronidazole) is necessary to prevent tubal damage and infertility. An IUCD should be removed once antibiotics have been started, since it will form a focus of infection. If neglected, a tubal abscess (pyosalpinx) or pelvic abscess develops with increasing pain, rigors and a tender mass. An abscess needs surgical drainage, but sometimes drains spontaneously into the rectum. Adhesions always form and generalized peritonitis never develops. Tubal cilia are damaged and infertility can occur even without total occlusion (which occurs in 75% of those with 3 or more episodes). Ectopic pregnancy is more common following salpingitis.

Chronic salpingitis
— recurrent salpingitis
— tuberculosis

The tubes become occluded, fibrous adhesions develop and the uterus is fixed in retroversion. The symptoms are:

— pain (congestive dysmenorrhoea, deep dyspareunia, low abdominal and back pain)
— menorrhagia
— discharge and low-grade fever
— bilateral tender adnexal masses

There is a history of previous attacks of salpingitis but laparoscopy may be necessary to differentiate if from endometriosis. Acute exacerbations are common and prolonged courses of rotating antibiotics are necessary. If it is causing chronic ill-health, hysterectomy and bilateral salpingectomy is the best treatment, conserving healthy ovarian tissue if possible.

Pelvic tuberculosis (always due to haematogenous spread) usually presents with infertility but can produce all the above symptoms. It is suspected if there is a history of contact, if the patient is a virgin or if there is no response to antibiotics. CXR, ESR and lymphocyte counts would be indicated but the definitive diagnosis is on histology of curettings. It is treated with rifampicin, isoniazid and ethambutol.

Pelvic mass   A lump in the pelvis is notoriously difficult to diagnose clinically. A malignant ovarian tumour is always a possibility. Ultrasound and laparoscopy may be indicated. The possibilities are:

— ovarian cyst or tumour
— fibroid (especially if pedunculated)
— bladder
— pregnancy (6–10 weeks)
— tubal pregnancy
— endometriosis (chocolate cysts)
— hydro/pyo-salpinx
— bowel (faeces, diverticular disease, carcinoma, Crohn's)
— pelvic kidney (very rare)
— haematocolpos (pubertal girls)

Fibroids   Fibroids are benign tumours of the uterine smooth muscle and are often multiple. They are more common in Africans. They can enlarge in pregnancy or on the pill. They regress after the menopause. They may grow inwards (submucus) or outwards (subserous) and are often symptomless.

Classically a woman over 35 who is either infertile or has not had a baby for many years, presents with menorrhagia. Occasionally they present as an abdominal lump or with pressure symptoms (frequency or swollen legs).

The hard, rounded lumps may be felt abdominally, and vaginally they move with the cervix. Ultrasound confirms the diagnosis and excludes an ovarian cyst. If small and symptomless, follow up 6-monthly. If large (16 weeks size), or causing symptoms, hysterectomy is the best treatment. Younger women may prefer myomectomy but this can be a long operation with risk of haemorrhage and, later, adhesions, and the fibroids tend to recur. Histology may show areas of degeneration (hyaline cystic, calcerous), or, very rarely, sarcomatous change.

In pregnancy fibroids often enlarge but normal labour is possible. Rarely, cervical fibroids occur and can obstruct labour. PPH is more common.

Red degeneration of a fibroid is usually only seen in pregnancy. It causes acute abdominal pain, fever and vomiting. Often the woman is known to have fibroids because of a previous scan. The important sign is a tender spot on the uterus, which moves with the uterus when the woman turns on her side, distinguishing it from appendicitis or torsion of an ovarian cyst. It is treated with strong analgesics. Surgery is avoided because the degenerating fibroid can bleed profusely. Torsion of a pedunculated fibroid presents like torsion of an ovarian cyst and requires laparotomy.

Hysterectomy   Most hysterectomies are performed for benign conditions. The proportions in 1975 in England and Wales were:

Menorrhagia — 33%
Fibroids   — 25%
Prolapse   — 12%
Unclassified — 23%
Malignancies — 7%

In 1981 63,560 hysterectomies were performed in England and Wales. Each GP is likely to be involved with counselling at least 2 women per year for the operation. There is a low mortality and morbidity from the operation. There is a wide regional variation in hysterectomy rates suggesting it is an operation affected to some extent by opinion or fashion.

Endometriosis   Endometriosis means ectopic endometrium, usually on the ovaries and in the pouch of Douglas, which probably gets implanted following retrograde menstruation. It bleeds at the time of menstruation, causing an intense fibrous reaction and dense adhesions. It can be symptomless even when extensive, but the typical clinical picture is of an infertile woman of 30–45 with:

— dysmenorrhoea
— dyspareunia
— menorrhagia
— tender retroverted uterus
— large tender ovaries (chocolate cysts)

Clinical diagnosis is notoriously difficult and laparoscopy is essential to distinguish endometriosis from chronic salpingitis. The tubes characteristically remain patent in endometriosis, and infertility is probably due to ovarian deposits preventing ovum release.

Endometriosis regresses in pregnancy (and after the menopause) and hormone treatment aims to produce a state of pseudo-pregnancy. Kisfner introduced combined oestrogen-progestogen treatment in 1958. The continuous use of a combined oral contraceptive pill can be used to relieve symptoms in mild endometriosis.

The treatment of choice is the more expensive *danazol* (Danol). 200–800 mg daily can be used. It is an anti-gonadotrophin and inhibits FSH and LH (flushes, sweats, reduced breast size). It is a derivative of testosterone (hence fluid retention, acne and sometimes virilization).

As endometriosis resolves, fertility improves and non-hormonal contraception should be used if pregnancy is not desired (the pill interferes with treatment). *Surgery* is also used:

— Small black deposits seen at laparotomy can be diathermied
— Ovarian cysts need to be excised if fertility is desired (they will not resolve on danazol)
— Widespread disease ('the frozen pelvis') in older women requires hysterectomy and BSO

— Adenomyosis (ectopic endometrium within the myometrium) causes menorrhagia and an enlarged tender uterus and usually requires hysterectomy

Ovarian cysts
— distension cysts (small)
— mucinous
— serous
— dermoid
— endometrial

1. Distension cysts are either:

— follicular (more common with clomiphene, Pergonal)
— luteal (can rupture and bleed)
— multiple luteal (mole)

They are small (less than 5 cm) and translucent if seen at laparoscopy. No treatment is needed, but follow-up examinations are necessary until they disappear.

2. Benign cysts are usually symptomless, but may present with abdominal swelling or discomfort or rarely with urinary retention if it incarcerates. Diagnosis is confirmed by scan. All cysts larger than 5 cm must be removed by cystectomy without tapping, because 15% are malignant. Near the menopause BSO and total hysterectomy can be performed.

Mechanical complications of torsion, rupture or haemorrhage into a cyst present as acute abdominal pain and require laparotomy.

3. In pregnancy there is an increased likelihood of torsion. Cysts are removed after 16 weeks, in case it is a corpus luteal cyst producing progesterone that is maintaining the pregnancy.

Ovarian cancer
— mucinous adenocarcinoma (cystic)
— serous adenocarcinoma (cystic)
— solid adenocarcinoma (primary or secondary)
— dysgerminoma (peak age 18, radio-sensitive)
— Granulosa cell (small and secretes hormones)

On average a GP will see one new case every 6 years. Prognosis depends more on spread than histology and survival is poor (overall 5YS is 30%) due to late presentation. 25% are bilateral. The peak age is 50–60 years and there is an increased incidence in the nulliparous and Social Class 1.

The main symptoms are:

— abdominal pains
— abdominal swelling (ascites)

but the condition is notoriously silent.

A postmenopausal woman with either an adnexal mass or ascites should be presumed to have a malignant ovarian tumour until proved otherwise. Signs suggestive of malignancy are:

— irregular mass
— bilateral mass
— ascites
— non-tender nodules in pouch of Douglas
— swollen leg (iliac vein compression)
— back pain (metastases)
— intestinal obstruction
— high urea (ureteric obstruction)
— shadows on CXR

Ultrasound confirms an ovarian mass, but if any pelvic lump is present, laparotomy is always indicated (even if malignant cells are seen in the ascitic fluid) for diagnosis and histology, staging and excision (Table 2).

Table 2 Stages of ovarian cancer

STAGE	SPREAD	TREATMENT	5YS (%) — FIGO
1a.	Ovary	Surgery	90
1b.	Both ovaries	Surgery	60
2.	Spread to pelvis	Surgery ± CT ± RT	40
3.	Spread to abdomen	Surgery ± CT ± RT	25
4.	Metastases	Surgery ± CT ± RT	15

CT = chemotherapy   RT = radiotherapy

Surgery of Stage 1a in a young woman involves oophorectomy and biopsy of the other ovary. Otherwise, surgery means total abdominal hysterectomy, BSO, omenectomy and debulking of any remaining tumour.

The menopause   The average age for cessation of periods in Britain is 50 with a range of 40–57 years. The problems are:

— irregular cycles
— contraception
— hot flushes, night sweats
— genital atrophy
— mood changes
— osteoporosis; atherosclerosis
— hormone replacement therapy (HRT)

1. Irregular cycles are common as the menopause approaches because falling oestrogen levels (follicular failure) no longer stimulate an LH surge and cycles become anovular. An interval of more than 6 months between bleeds is an indication for curettage to exclude endometrial carcinoma. If curettage is normal but a second episode of bleeding after 6 months of amenorrhoea occurs, some specialists advice hysterectomy. With heavy bleeding check FBC and thyroid function. After a curettage has excluded abnormality treat with mefanamic acid or cyclic progestogens or danazol for heavy bleeding.
2. Barrier methods, the POP or the IUCD can be stopped

12 months after the last period. If there is amenorrhoea and hot flushes, fertility can be assumed to have ceased.

The POP is very effective at this stage of relatively low fertility (failure rate about 0.5%) and it often helps hot flushes. However, if breakthrough bleeding occurs, curettage is necessary.

In the absence of smoking, obesity or hypertension, it may become acceptable to continue the Combined Pill up to the menopause. HRT is *not* contraceptive.

3. Vasomotor instability causes hot flushes with sweating and palpitations. They occur in 75% but only about 15% request treatment.

They last a few minutes and can occur up to 50 times a day. They may last a few months or 5 years or more, but unlike genital atrophy they eventually cease even without treatment. They are probably due to high FSH levels and respond within days to HRT.

4. Genital tract atrophy predisposes to:

— atrophic vaginitis
— prolapse
— stress incontinence

Atrophic vaginitis is common, causing soreness, dysuria, dyspareunia and eventually shrinkage of the introitus.

There may be a blood-stained discharge (often sterile but there is a tendency to bacterial infection because of loss of protective acidity, therefore take swabs).

It is treated with topical oestrogens (e.g. stilboestrol cream) or oral oestrogens (e.g. Premarin 0.625 mg daily) or by longterm HRT.

5. Mood changes, headaches, insomnia, irritability and depression are common around the menopause. Often they are due to simultaneous stress associated with family and job, together with feelings of loss of attractiveness and low self-esteem. Oestrogen deficiency can cause mood changes, however, that respond dramatically to HRT. Clinical depression is better treated with a tricyclic antidepressant.

6. There is an increased incidence of osteoporotic fractures (neck of femur, wrist, vertebra) and of myocardial infarctions (serum cholesterol and triglycerides become elevated) after the menopause. This can be used as an argument for prolonged HRT.

7. Hormone replacement therapy (HRT) is indicated for:

— atrophic vagingitis
— hot flushes

The best preparations are those combining a natural oestrogen (said to have fewer side effects) for 11 days and an oestrogen and progesterone for the next 10 days (e.g. Cyclo-Progynova). There is evidence that the progesterone protects the woman from endometrial carcinoma, which is associated with prolonged unopposed oestrogen.

Withdrawal bleeds occur, because it is given clinically for three weeks out of four to prevent endometrial build up and irregular bleeding. Any bleeding between these regular withdrawal bleeds indicates curettage to exclude carcinoma. HRT is not a contraceptive (the dose of oestrogen is only equivalent to about 10 μg of the synthetic oestrogen used in the Combined Pill)

HRT is felt to be contraindicated with:

— thrombo-embolism (or a trial fibrillation)
— active liver disease
— carcinoma (breast, endometrium, ovary)

HRT should not be started if bleeding is already irregular. Several factors may combine to contra-indicate it (e.g. an obese, hypertensive smoker). Some say HRT can be used indefinitely in women who have had a hysterectomy, when it is safe to use oestrogens alone (e.g. ethinyl-oestradiol 0.01 mg daily or BD). It may cause nausea and breast tenderness initially. If contraindicated, consider the POP (also contraceptive), norethisterone, clonidine or Bellergal.

Endometrical carcinoma

On average a GP will see one new case every 7 years. Endometrial carcinoma is an adenocarcinoma that usually occurs in postmenopausal women. The peak age is 60 years and 50% are nulliparous. It is thought to be due to prolonged unopposed oestrogen stimulation because:

1. In experimental animals, high-dose oestrogens cause hyperplasia that is premalignant
2. It was seen more commonly in women on prolonged hormone replacement using oestrogens only
3. There is sometimes a history of dysfunctional bleeding and late menopause, suggesting high oestrogen levels
4. There is evidence that these women have an increased peripheral conversion of androstendione to oestrone

The classical symptom is *post-menopausal bleeding*. Any bleeding 6 months after the periods have stopped merits investigation. It should also be suspected with irregular premenopausal bleeding or if there is a persistent watery discharge. There are usually no signs and the uterus is not enlarged. Diagnostic curettage is performed and repeated in 3 months if negative. Fractional curettage means attempting to take separate curettings from the body and cervix to help with staging. The over all 5YS is 65% (the thick uterine muscle makes local spread slower than in carcinoma of the cervix (Table 3).

Treatment is by preoperative intracavity radium followed by extended hysterectomy (i.e. including a cuff of vagina where recurrence occurs most commonly) and BSO.

Radiotherapy alone is only used in patients unfit for surgery.

Table 3 Stages of endometrial carcinoma

STAGE	SITE	5YS (%)
1.	Body	90
2.	Cervix	50
3.	Vagina/parametrium	Poor
4.	Bladder, rectum, metastases	Poor

Metastatic disease is treated with high dose progesterone e.g. Medroxyprogesterone 250 mg daily (fluid retention) which can produce remission. It is most useful in well differentiated, slow-growing tumours.

Prolapse   The main causes are childbirth, menopausal atrophy and raised intra-abdominal pressure (e.g. obesity, smokers cough or rarely ascites or a large ovarian cyst). It is sometimes seen in the nulliparous however, presumably due to congenital weakness of the main uterine supports (transverse cervical and utero-sacral ligaments), which normally 'anchor' the cervix in the middle of the pelvis.

The diagnostic pointer in the history is that all the symptoms are *worse on standing* and relieved by lying down:

— something coming down
— backache
— stress incontinence

The patient may also complain of difficulty voiding urine or defaecating, which they relieve by digital pressure on either the anterior or posterior vaginal wall.

The diagnosis is confirmed by examination. Prolapsed vaginal wall (cystocele, rectocele) can occur without uterine descent but prolapse of the uterus (descent of the cervix below the level of the ischial spines) rarely occurs alone.

The left lateral position using a Sim's speculum to retract the perineum is the best position to demonstrate a urethrocele (lower third) or cystocele. As the woman bears down, descent of the cervix may also be visible; a finger in the rectum pressed anteriorly will demonstrate a rectocele. Uterine descent is best assessed by bimanual examination.

Treatment can be by:

1. A polyethylene ring pessary (rubber ones can cause vaginitis). This is inserted like a diaphragm and should be changed every 4 months. There is often an element of atrophy, when oestrogens are helpful. The woman should be encouraged to lose weight and stop smoking.

A pessary can be used if the woman is unfit for surgery or is awaiting surgery. A pessary can also be used in early pregnancy if there is any prolapse and removed at 16 weeks when the uterus becomes abdominal.

2. Vaginal hysterectomy and repair (i.e. including anterior colporraphy and posterior colpoperineorraphy) is usually the treatment of choice, especially if the woman has heavy periods or is post-menopausal. The utero-sacral ligaments are sewn together to prevent a subsequent enterocele.

It involves a 10-day admission. A brown discharge occurs for 2–3 weeks afterwards, sometimes with strands of suture material. Heavy lifting and intercourse are forbidden for 6 weeks. The vagina is slightly shortened but soon lengthens with regular intercourse.

3. The alternative operation is the Manchester repair (amputation of the cervix and suturing together the transverse cervical ligaments) following which child-birth is still possible.

Urinary incontinence

It is important to distinguish between *stress* incontinence which can be treated surgically and *urge* incontinence which cannot.

1. Stress incontinence

Stress incontinence means troublesome involuntary leakage of urine when the intra-abdominal pressure is raised — e.g. coughing, sneezing, laughing, running and lifting. It occurs to a slight degree in 10% of women who have had children. The classic finding on examination is a cystocele and incontinence on coughing that can be prevented by digital para-urethral pressure (Bonney's test).

However stress incontinence can occur in the absence of these signs. If cystometry is performed it is normal apart from a low urethral closing pressure when the patient tries to squeeze the device.

The essential abnormality is descent of the upper urethra through the pelvic floor (levator ani) so that it is no longer compressed with the bladder when intra-abdominal pressure rises.

Pubococcygeus (part of levator ani) is lax and no longer pulls the upper urethra forward, so that the posterior vesico-urethral angle is characteristically flat on a micturating cystogram (although this can be seen without any stress incontinence).

The voluntary sphincter (the compressor urethrae, part of the deep perineal muscle) maintains continence at other times.

Treatment

a) Pelvic floor exercises can relieve stress incontinence. The woman is taught how to elevate the perineum and 'contract the vagina', as if trying to prevent her bowels moving. This sensation can be demonstrated on examination by teaching her to pull up the perineum against the examining fingers or to squeeze the fingers or alternatively by one or two sessions of faradic stimulation by the physiotherapist.

If the woman is diligent with these exercises, they do work; they should be advised for all women after childbirth to prevent later stress incontinence.

b) A simple anterior repair (colporraphy) relieves symptoms in 70%. If it fails, transabdominal colposuspension operations can be tried, e.g. stitching the bladder to the back of the pubis (Marshall and Marchetti) or by a suburethral sling of fascia stitched to the rectus sheath (Aldridge).

Following these operations a suprapubic catheter is needed for several days because micturition is obviously difficult. Elective section is usually advised for future pregnancies.

2. Urge incontinence   Urge incontinence means the sudden desire to void rapidly followed by incontinence. There is usually also frequency. It is due to an irritable bladder and is often difficult to treat. Surgery is no help and tends to make it worse.

It is diagnosed by cystometry which shows detrusor contractions on minor pressure rises or even changes in posture. Management may include:

— exclude a UTI
— cystoscopy and IVU (stone or tumour?)
— cystometry (to confirm diagnosis)
— drugs are some help in 50%. Either anticholinergics like emepronium bromide (Cetiprin) 200 mg q.d.s. or antispasmodics like flavoxate (Urispas) 200 mg q.d.s.
— hydrostatic dilatation under epidural. This helps about 80% initially but only about 50% by one year.
— remember rare causes of urge incontinence — multiple sclerosis or cord compression. It can also occur in:

   — pregnancy
   — large ovarian cyst
   — salpingitis; endometriosis

Continuous dribbling occurs with:

— vesico-vaginal fistula (radiotherapy, carcinoma or prolonged obstructed labour)
— retention with overflow, when the bladder will be palpable. This is usually due to diabetic neuropathy

Backache   Gynaecological backache is continuous, bilateral aching, below the iliac crests, quite unlike lumbar root pain (sudden onset, worse on movement, radiation, tenderness).
Consider:

— prolapse
— retroversion
— endometriosis
— chronic salpingitis
— carcinoma of the cervix
— vertebral metastases

Retroversion is common and rarely causes backache. A

Hodge pessary can be inserted to hold the uterus anteverted for a few weeks. If this relieves the symptoms then ventro-suspension (suturing the round ligaments to the rectus sheath) may be justified and can be performed at laparoscopy.

In endometriosis and chronic salpingitis the pain tends to be worse before periods and there will be other symptoms (dyspareunia, menorrhagia and discharge). Laparoscopy is indicated.

Family Planning

The ideal contraceptive (which does not exist) would have the following characteristics:

— 100% effective
— No danger
— No nuisance
— 100% reversible by simple procedure
— Independent of intercourse
— Not relying on user motivation
— Cheap and easy to distribute
— Pre-fertilization in action
— Used by or visible to the woman
— Independent of the medical profession
— One or more good effects (e.g. reduced risk of STDs)

Failure rates The figures in Table 4 for % failure rates per year are useful when discussing the relative effectiveness of each method. The figures can only be approximate for a given couple because effectiveness depends upon how the method is used. Some couples use withdrawal as a successful method of contraception, others get pregnant with the diaphragm or pill because they use them incorrectly. Furthermore, failure rate will be influenced by fertility, sexual activity and the length of time that the particular method has been used.

Table 4 Failure rates for different contraceptive methods

Method	% Failures/year
Sterilization	0.1
Combined Pill	0.1
POP	2
Medroxy-progesterone	2
IUCD	2
Diaphragm	3
Vaginal sponge	3–6
Sheath	4
Spermicide alone	10
Natural (mucus and temperature)	12
Withdrawal	16
Natural (calendar alone)	24

Contraceptive usage In the UK in 1980, in millions:

Pills	3.0
Sheath	2.8

Withdrawal	0.7
IUCD	0.5
Diaphragm	0.2

Before 1960 birth control meant barrier methods, withdrawal or abstinence. The pill, the IUCD, injectables, sterilization and termination were basically unavailable.

Questions about contraception were included in the 1983 *General Household Survey*. Three quarters of all women aged 18–44 were using contraception (one half of those aged 18–19 and four fifths of those aged 25–39). The proportion relying on each method were:

Pill	—	28%
Sterilization	—	22%
Condom	—	13%
Withdrawal	—	4%
Cap	—	1%
Chemicals	—	1%

General advice

1. The doctor must be able to compare the benefits and risks of the different methods of contraception but should never dictate which method has to be used. It is a personal matter for the couple to decide, having understood the facts with the help of a doctor.

2. It is important to get the risks of contraception into perspective. The figures in Table 5 (death rates per 100 000 users, live births or abortions) are approximations to give an idea of the relative risks of contraception compared to pregnancy. In fact the risks rise steadily with age. Note that the figures do not include morbidity (pain, menorrhagia, infection are increased with the IUCD).

Table 5 Death rates for various forms of contraception and for pregnancy (per 100 000 users)

	Under 35	Over 35
IUCD	1	1
Legal termination	2	3
Pill	2	12
Pill and smoking	8	40
Pregnancy	15	50

3. *The Combined Pill* is usually the method of choice, provided there are no contraindications (thrombosis, liver disease, migraine) and can probably safely be continued after 35 provided the woman is a non-smoker, normotensive and not obese.

4. *The POP* is less effective when fertility is high but can safely be used if the Combined Pill is contraindicated. It is also used during breast feeding as it does not supress lactation. Breakthrough bleeding is a common problem.

5. *The IUCD* is ideal when responsibility or motivation for contraception is lacking. It is mainly used in the multip who is spacing her family or has completed her family and does not want the Pill or sterilization. It is not suitable for nullips (expulsion, failure and infection rates are high).

6. *The sheath* is widely used and very safe if used every time with a spermicide. No medical supervision is needed. It spoils the spontaneity of sex for some couples.

7. *The diaphragm* with spermicide is a very effective method if used properly. It requires fitting and initial instruction and a lot of women think of it as messy and off-putting. However it can be inserted several hours before intercourse (or ideally routinely every night) and neither partner can feel it during intercourse. It also has no side-effects (except possibly mechanical cystitis if it is too large).

8. *Natural methods* can be very effective if used consistently by well-motivated, intelligent couples. The ideal is to use a combination of the calendar methods, temperature chart and cervical mucus examination (Billing's method) to predict when ovulation occurs and to avoid coitus for 4 days either side. However, many couples use the method incorrectly and also practice withdrawal during the fertile days, making for a high failure rate.

9. *Sterilization* is the ideal method of contraception for the couple who have completed their family, have a stable relationship, are sure they do not want any more children and have several years of potential fertility ahead of them. It should be considered irreversible.

10. *Withdrawal* is still commonly used as a method of contraception, often just called 'being careful'. If a couple are happy to use the method and do so effectively then it is a good method of contraception for them. They are unlikely to start using barrier methods if they find them distasteful and have always found withdrawal to be effective. They might be persuaded to use a spermicide alone.

11. *Post-coital douching* is of no contraceptive value because sperms enter the cervical canal within seconds of ejaculation. Douching is unnecessary for hygienic purposes and indeed can predispose to vaginal infection.

12. Women attending *Family Planning Clinics* often feel able to discuss anxieties or embarrassing problems. It is also a good time for health education and screening. Apart from contraceptive advice the clinics undertake:

— cervical smears
— teaching self breast examination
— detection of symptomless venereal disease
— psychosexual counselling

13. In developing countries, *prolonged lactation* could be more encouraged for its contraceptive value. It is not completely

reliable for any individual but markedly reduces the fertility of a community.

The Combined Pill The combined oral contraceptive pill has been on the market since 1960. There are 65 million users worldwide. All varieties contain either ethinyloestradiol (EE) or mestranol (which is metabolized to ethinyloestradiol) together with a derivative of 19 nor-testosterone (norethisterone, L-norgestrel or ethynodiol, lynoestrenol or desogestrel). L-norgestrel and desogestrel are, 5 × more potent than the others.

They cause:

1. Inhibition of ovulation, by negative feedback on FSH and LH. Occasional ovulation can occur with the 20 μg oestrogen formulations.

2. Replacement of endogenous oestrogen and progesterone causing:

— viscid cervical mucus
— atrophic endometrium with reduced risk of implantation (less marked with phasic pills).

It is useful to understand and use a few formulations:

1. First choice should be a pill with low doses of both oestrogen and progestogen (to minimize side-effects) e.g.:

— Brevinor (EE 35 μg; Norethisterone 0.5 mg)
— Marvelon (EE 30 μg; Desogestrel 0.15 mg)

Side effects are rare with low dose pills. There is no good evidence that changing the oestrogen-progestogen balance relieves symptoms thought to be due to high oestrogens (fluid retention, nausea, PMS, vaginal discharge) or high progestogens (acne, hirsutism, dry vagina, loss of libido, depression). If symptoms persist for more than 2 months change to another pill with low doses of both hormones. Usually the only reason for changing to a pill with higher doses is poor cycle control. If side effects are troublesome a POP should be considered.

2. The triphasic pill (e.g. Trinordiol) aims to mimic physiological hormone changes and to keep dosage and side-effects to a minimum. It is effective but expensive. It consists of:

No. of tablets	6	5	10 (21 days)
EE	30	40	30
Norgestrel	50	75	125

It tends to be tried if other pills cause side-effects.

3. 50 g ethinyloestrodiol (e.g. Minovlar) is necessary if the woman is taking drugs that are enzyme inducers (rifampicin, phenobarbitone, phenytoin, carbamazepine), or if the woman gets troublesome breakthrough bleeding (spotting) with lower dose pills.

4. The progestogen-dominant brands (Conova 30, Eugynon

30 and 50, Ovran 30 and Ovran) are best avoided because they lower levels of HDL-cholesterol and favour atherosclerosis and may account for the association of the pill with arterial disease.

Prescribing the Combined Pill

1. Discuss contraceptive needs in general. Occasionally another method is more suitable. A request for the pill may be her way of presenting with an emotional problem.

2. *Past history* — exclude contraindications. Drugs (rifampicin, phenobarbitone, phenytoin or carbamazepine. A higher dose of warfarin or insulin may be necessary). The Combined Pill may precipitate diabetes if there is a strong family history. Contact lenses may need changing (corneal fluid retention). Primary dysmenorrhoea will usually be relieved by the pill.

3. Women on the pill should be strongly advised against *smoking*. It should not be prescribed to smokers over 35. The risks (still largely unknown) should be discussed but so should the benefits (effectively 100% protection, less dysmenorrhoea, less fibroadenosis of the breast).

4. *Explain how to use the pill*:

— Start Day 1 and it is safe immediately
— Establish a routine (e.g. bedtime)
— During the 7 pill-free days intercourse is still safe and the 'period' will be lighter than usual
— If the pill is forgotten by less than 12 hours — safe
— If the pill is forgotten by more than 12 hours — unsafe. Take it anyway but use a sheath for 14 days.
— If after taking the pill vomiting (within 2 hours) or diarrhoea (within 12 hours) occur — unsafe, so use a sheath for 14 days.
— *Minor side effects* (nausea, breast tenderness, headache) are common at first but wear off after 2–3 cycles
— If bleeding occurs between periods or no 'period' (withdrawal bleed) occurs, do not stop the pill — if concerned make an appointment to see the doctor.

N.B. Pills forgotten at the beginning or end of the packet are probably the most likely to result in 'method failure', because the pill-free interval is increased, and pituitary inhibition is therefore less.

5. *Breakthrough bleeding* between periods can occur on the lower dose pills — especially if the woman takes ampicillin. If persistent a pill with a higher dose of progestogen can be tried.

6. *Absent withdrawal bleeds* are harmless and unrelated to post-pill amenorrhoea. If there is a possibility of pregnancy (i.e. the woman is not certain that she has taken the pill correctly) it must be excluded. If she is pregnant and has been taking the pill, she can be reassured that there is no evidence of increased fetal abnormality.

Having no monthly bleed worries some women ('what

happens to the blood?'). Increasing the dose of oestrogen will make withdrawal bleeds return.

7. *See in 6 weeks* (middle of second packet) to discuss any problems. Then see every 6 months to check:

— BP
— weight
— urine for sugar

All sexually-active women should have *cervical smears*. The first one can be delayed until the 6-monthly check if the woman is nervous. Repeat at 1 year then every 3 years (ideally for ever). 50% of women on the pill develop an erosion, which only needs cryocautery if symptomatic. Also check rubella status.

8. When prescribing ampicillin remember:

— the pill may not be as effective (use a sheath)
— it can precipitate candidiasis

9. The should be stopped at least a month before elective surgery and not recommenced until 2 months afterwards. It should also be stopped if the woman becomes immobilized (e.g. fractures).

10. Form FP1001 should be completed every 12 months to claim for payment for contraceptive advice, prescription of pills or diaphragms or follow-up care. Form FP1003 is used for temporary residents.

Contraindications to the
Combined Pill

— age over 45
— obesity (> 50% ideal weight)
— family History of CVS disease (in first degree relative under 45).
— hyperlipidaemia (atherogenic profile)
— heavy smoker (> 50 cigarettes per day)
— actual or possible pregnancy
— undiagnosed genital bleeding
— any severe condition worsened by pregnancy (e.g. chorea, otosclerosis)
— DVT or pulmonary embolus
— liver disease (active)
— cholestasis in pregnancy
— hypertension (above 160/100).
— migraine or TIAs
— heart disease (valvular or ischaemic)
— polycythaemia or sickle cell anaemia
— carcinoma of breast or cervix
— porphyria
— hydatidiform mole (recent)
— hyperprolactinaemia (tumour may enlarge)
— Crohns disease
— benign intracranial hypertension

N.B. A history of irregular periods does not contraindicate the pill, since post-pill amenorrhoea is treatable with clomiphene. Varicose veins are not a contraindication, although the pill should be stopped before veins are injected.

Complications of the
Combined Pill

1. *Cardiovascular accidents* (venous and arterial). The increased mortality from the pill, highlighted by the 1977 RCGP study, was due to myocardial infarction, stroke, subarachnoid arterial embolus (i.e. arterial complications).

23 000 pill-users were compared with 23 000 non-users. 55 'ever users' died, compared to 10 'never users', a five fold increase in risk.

Factors that contribute to the increased risk seem to be:

— smoking
— age over 35
— obesity
— hypertension
— diabetes
— hypercholesterolaemia

In a 1981 report on the study it emerged that duration of pill-use does not increase the risk (e.g. a woman on the pill for 10 years is at no more risk than after 1 year) provided the pill is stopped in those who develop hypertension.

Women who smoke face by far the greatest hazard. The death rate from cardiovascular disease in women aged 25–34 on the pill is 4.4/100 000 in non-smokers and 14.2/100 000 in smokers. Women who do not smoke, particularly under 35, are hardly any more at risk than a non-user, and are far less at risk than if they became pregnant.

The overall risk remains unknown, and in fact mortality rates for women between 1950 and 1976 decreased more than did those for men.

Indications for stopping the pill:

— Emergence of a contraindication
— Change in age or smoking habit
— Diastolic pressure >95 (sustained)
— Jaundice
— Elective major surgery (1 month before)
— Varicose vein surgery (1 month before)
— Longterm immobilization
— Migraine (with focal features)
— Swollen calf (venogram)
— Suspected pulmonary embolisms
— Transient weakness (?CVA)
— Disturbed speech (?CVA)
— Visual disturbances (?TIA)
— A collapse (?TIA)

2. *Hypertension* develops in 5% of pill users after 5 years. The risk is increased if there is a history of hypertension in pregnancy, renal disease or a strong family history.

If the BP rises above 160 systolic or 95 diastolic the pill should be stopped. If the BP fails to return to normal within 6 months it needs investigating.

No woman with unexplained hypertension should take the pill, and BP should be monitored every 6 months in all women on the pill.

3. *Fertility* is not impaired by the pill, although women who stop the pill can suffer a delay of a few months before the restoration of normal fertility.

Post-pill amenorrhoea needs full investigation but nearly always responds to clomiphene.

4. *The incidence of gallstones* is slightly increased after 3 years on the pill.

5. *The metabolic effects* of the pill are:

— increased cholesterol
— increased triglycerides
— increased renin substrate (hyptertension)
— increased platelet stickiness
— enzyme induction

6. *Drug interactions*. Rifampicin, phenobarbitone, phenytoin and carbamazepine are enzyme-inducers and lower the plasma levels of EE. Women on these drugs should be prescribed a 50 μg pill.

Ampicillin can lower the oestrogen levels (probably by decreasing gut flora that deconjugate EE prior to reabsorbtion). Irregular bleeding may occur and pregnancies have been reported.

Higher doses of insulin or warfarin may be needed.

7. *Depression* due to the pill sometimes responds to supplements of pyridoxine, 100 mg daily.

The combined pill can be used to treat:

— dysmenorrhoea
— ovulation pain
— menorrhagia
— endometriosis
— functional ovarian cysts
— regulation of periods (after disease excluded)

There is a decreased incidence of benign breast disease, ectopic pregnancies and carcinoma of the ovary and endometrium in women on the combined pill.

Note: The 1985 House of Lords ruling means it is legal to prescribe the pill to girls under 16 without their parent's consent.

The progesterone-only pill (POP)

In order of increasing strength:

		Pills per packet
Microval (L-norgestrel 30 mcg)	—	35
Norgeston (L-norgestrel 30 mcg)	—	35
Neogest (L-norgestrel 77.5 mcg)	—	35
Micronor (norethisterone 350 mcg)	—	28
Noriday (norethisterone 350 mcg)	—	28
Femulen (ethynodiol 500 mcg)	—	28

The POP or 'mini-pill' has a failure rate of 2% per year but this falls with age. Its main action is on cervical mucus (an 'oral barrier method') but it also makes the endometrium unreceptive and in some women inhibits ovulation.

It is contraindicated with a history of ectopics (? slows tubal motility and increases the risk) or in those with an increased risk of ectopics e.g. with a history of pelvic inflammatory disease or following tubal surgery. Pregnancies occuring on the POP are more likely to be ectopic. There is no evidence of a tendency to thrombosis. The POP has no major undesirable side-effects. It is contra-indicated in:

— previous ectopic pregnancy
— undiagnosed vaginal bleeding
— severe arterial disease (past or present)
— hypertriglyceridaemia
— hydatidiform mole (until HCG normal)
— carcinoma of the breast (theoretical risk)

Enzyme inducers (rifampiam, anticonvulsants) will reduce the contraceptive efficacy.

Uses

1. Contraception during lactation. The POP does not suppress lactation (although the 30 μg oestrogen pills probably do not suppress lactation either).

It is excreted in minute amounts in breast milk but has no known adverse effects on the baby.

Change to the Combined Pill on the first day of a period, once breast feeding is no longer required.

2. Contraception for women with troublesome oestrogenic side-effects from the Combined Pill:

— Fluid retention, weight gain
— headache
— Chloasma

3. The POP can be used if the Combined Pill is contra-indicated by:

— migraine
— thrombosis, embolus
— liver disease
— hypertension

— diabetes
— over 35 and a smoker

High density lipoprotein levels are not significantly altered by the POP. When the POP is prescribed for patients who have become hypertensive on the combined pill the BP usually drops to normal.

4. In diabetics the POP may reduce the risks of arterial disease and of accelerating retiropathy.

5. For older women, the POP can be a very suitable method of contraception. A problem is knowing when the menopause is reached. Elevated FSH is probably diagnostic. Hot flushes or amenorrhoea may occur, when the POP should be stopped and alternative methods used for at least a year.

Instructions

1. Take one tablet every day. A packet lasts 6 weeks. Start on Day 1 of a period and use a sheath for 14 days while the effect builds up. The ideal time to take it is 6 pm since the peak action occurs after about 5 hours. Stress that the POP must be taken at the same time every day — if more than 3 hours late on any day use sheath for 14 days.

If changing from the Combined Pill to the POP, start the day after the last pill.

2. Nausea, breast tenderness and breakthrough bleeding are common for the first packet but usually settle down.

3. If after taking the pill, vomiting (within 2 hours) or diarrhoea (within 12 hours) occur, take another pill.

Problems

1. It has a 2% failure rate per year in younger women.

2. It needs to be taken very accurately.

3. Irregular breakthrough bleeding often occurs and is the commonest reason for not liking the POP. It may be less on a higher dose (e.g. Femulen)

4. Missed periods. If there is a good chance of pregnancy stop the POP (since the effect on the fetus is unknown). If pregnancy is excluded (examine and send urine test), it means that the woman has had an anovular cycle and this low dose of hormone is inhibiting ovulation, making her extra-safe. It probably means she has an increased chance of post-pill amenorrhoea, (reversible with clomiphene).

5. Luteal cysts and abdominal pains occur occasionally.

6. Increased incidence of ectopics (0.1% of users).

Injectables

The usual drug is medroxyprogesterone (Depo-Provera) 150 mg i.m. every 3 months. An alternative is norethisterone oenanthate (Noristerat, Norigest) 200 mg (1 ml) i.m. every 8 weeks.

They are simple and highly effective but remain controversial. Effectiveness is probably even higher than the combined pill. The only indications in this country are:

1. with rubella vaccine
2. post vasectomy
3. Sickle cell disease. The disease is actually improved with increased Hb and reduced crises.

They must be given on Day 1–3 of bleeding to be effective for that cycle.

The problems are:

1. Irregular breakthrough bleeding between periods
2. They can induce amenorrhoea and impaired fertility for up to a year afterwards.
3. Weight gain
4. Possible carcinogenicity. This relates to breast nodules in beagle dogs, but so far human studies have not verified this.

The Intra-Uterine Device (IUCD)

The IUCD is used by 8% of women in the UK needing contraception (half a million users). The failure rate is about 2% per year. A noticeable decline in failure rates is seen with increasing duration of use. The following types can be prescribed (on an FP10):

— Lippes loop (90% need size C)
— Copper-7
— Copper-T
— Multiload

The inert devices (Lippes loop) are larger and less likely to be expelled, and possibly slightly more effective, but they tend to cause more problems with pain and bleeding. It is safe to leave them *in situ* for many years but some doctors argue that they ought to be changed every 4 years to prevent them getting embedded (when curettage may be necessary to remove them). They are radio-opaque. They cause a sterile endometrial inflammation unsuitable for implantation (?leucocytes engulf ovum).

The copper-bearing devices (Copper-7, Copper-T, Multiload) are smaller and easier to insert but need changing every 3 years. They tend to cause less problems of pain and bleeding. Copper is toxic to gametes.

If a woman has always been happy with a particular IUCD, it is sensible to insert the same type. Which coil is used is less important than the skill of the operator in:

— measuring the uterine cavity with a sound
— selecting the correct size
— inserting the IUCD correctly

The Multiload (one size) is probably the best first choice because it has low rates of perforation, expulsion, pain and bleeding. It also has the finest threads and can be tried if the man complains of feeling the thread. It is also relatively easy to insert.

The Copper-7 (Gravigard) is used for nullips as it has the narrowest introducer. A Minigravigard is also available.

Expensive devices (not prescribable on FP10): the Novagard (flexible T-shaped device using copper wire round a silver core) and the Progestasert (releases 65 μg of progesterone daily for 365 days and therefore must be changed every year. It can be tried if other IUCD's cause dysmnenorrhoea).

The method of insertion is slightly different for each type and needs to be taught and practised.

Advantages of the IUCD	— useful for the forgetful or if the pill is contraindicated

Advantages of the IUCD
— useful for the forgetful or if the pill is contraindicated
— long-term protection; more effective than barrier methods
— local action with no metabolic effects
— immediate action that is immediately reversible
— no day-to-day motivation needed (although high motivation is needed to have it inserted) and positive action needed to reverse it
— no supplies needed
— does not spoil the spontaneity of sex
— can be used when breast-feeding
— can be used for post-coital contraception (within 5 days)
— low mortality rate (and no evidence of increased endometrial carcinoma)
— relatively inexpensive

Indications   The IUCD is ideal when responsibility or motivation for contraception is lacking. It is suitable for the multip who is spacing her family or who has completed her family and does not want the pill or sterilization. It is least suitable for the nullip because insertion through the narrow cervix can be difficult (cervical shock) and because there are increased risks of:

— expulsion (irritable uterus)
— infection (4% in the first year) and subsequent infertility
— failure (4% per year)

Contraindications
— nullip who will accept another method
— pregnancy
— heavy or irregular bleeding
— dysmenorrhoea
— pelvic infection (within previous 6 months)
— previous ectopic pregnancy
— distorted cavity (large fibroids, bicornuate)
— cavity less than 5.5 cm (nullip)
— specific allergy to copper

Valvular heart disease is a relative contraindication but an IUCD can be fitted under antibiotic cover. A uterine scar is not a contraindication but a device with a low perforation rate (e.g. Multiload) should be used. An erosion is not a contraindication.

Insertion of the IUCD

This is best performed at the time of a period (as is removal) because:

1. pregnancy is excluded
2. the cervix is more dilated and softer
3. any bleeding will be masked by the period

An IUCD should not be inserted or removed (OR CHANGED, in case the second one won't go in) in the luteal half of the cycle when pregnancy is possible. However it can be deliberately inserted up to 5 days after unprotected intercourse as an effective form of post-coital contraception.

An IUCD can also be inserted at the time of termination. They are sometimes inserted immediately after childbirth or even caesarian section but there are 3 problems with this:

— high risk of perforation
— high expulsion rate
— possibility of confusing the diagnosis of postpartum harmorrhage

and it is best to wait until the 6-week postnatal check.

Choice of IUCD

In general copper devices have fewer side-effects than inert devices. Smaller devices (e.g. Minigravigard, Nova T) are best for the small nulliparous uterus. Larger devices e.g. Copper T, Multiload) are better suited to the larger parous uterus.

Method of insertion

1. Bimanual for position of uterus (anteverted or retroverted) to exclude pregnancy and screen for ovarian masses.
2. Smear if needed (screening)
3. Swab cervix with antiseptic
4. Apply tenaculum forceps to steady the cervix
5. Pass a sound
6. Insert IUCD of correct size using no touch technique
7. Repass the sound to check IUCD is not lying in the cervical canal (if it is, remove and replace)
8. The woman should rest for 10–20 minutes
9. (Sign FP1002)

N.B. During insertion painful traction or dilatation of the cervix can cause profound bradycardia and even unconsciousness (*cervical shock*). A Brook airway and 0.6 mg of atropine must always be at hand. If the IUCD has already been inserted it should be left. If the woman has severe pain on insertion she should remain horizontal for 5–10 minutes after the procedure. It is most likely to occur if:

— Nullip
— anxious and tense
— previous cervical surgery
— prolonged pill (cervix closes tight)

The following points must be explained:

1. Continue to use alternative contraception for the first 6 weeks (when expulsion rate is highest). The woman is seen again at 6 weeks to check the position. In the meantime she should check the threads every week. Most women say they cannot feel them but it is still worthwhile checking that the device is not palpable (i.e. lying in the canal).

2. Tampons can be used provided the threads are checked when one is removed. Intercourse can be resumed immediately.

3. Most women get crampy pains for 2 or 3 days after insertion and should be warned of this. It is more likely if insertion was painful and then Buscopan can be provided.

4. Some irregular spotting often occurs throughout the first cycle. The periods, particularly the first two or three, will be heavier. The normal discharge tends to get a bit heavier.

5. Annual follow-up is necessary for a smear (which will also pick up any actinomycosis) and to exclude anaemia if the IUCD causes heavy periods.

Problems of the IUCD

1. Heavy periods
2. Pain
3. Infection
4. Expulsion
5. Perforation
6. Pregnancy
7. Lost threads

1. *Heavy periods.* 10% request removal in the first year because of heavy periods. The smaller devices tend to double blood-loss, the larger inert devices to treble blood-loss. The first few cycles after insertion tend to be the heaviest, and some intermenstrual spotting may occur for the first cycle. After this any intermenstrual bleeding should not be ascribed to the IUCD (except for the Progestasert which does cause breakthrough bleeding).

A prostaglandin inhibitor or epsikapron can be used to decrease blood-loss, but most women prefer to try a smaller device or another method altogether.

2. *Colicky pains* are common for a few days after insertion. If they are persistent it suggests that the device is lying partially in the cervical canal, in which case it should be removed and another one correctly inserted.

Continuous pain in a woman with an IUCD may be due to:

— perforation
— infection
— ectopic

3. *Infection* is potentially the most serious complication of the IUCD. The normal uterine cavity is sterile but with an IUCD *in situ* it is not. Acute salpingitis occurs three times

more commonly in IUCD-users (about 2% of users per year) but is particularly common:

— shortly after insertion
— in the nullip

and increases the chances of subsequent ectopic pregnancy or fertility.

If infection develops (discharge, fever, pain) take swabs and start broad spectrum antibiotics, e.g. amoxycillin plus metronidazole. Removal of the IUCD is only necessary if there is no response after 2–3 days.

4. *Expulsion*. About 10% are expelled in the first year, mainly in the first few months. This usually causes colicky pain, but occasionally it is unnoticed and then contributes to the pregnancy rate. A device with a lower expulsion rate (Multiload, Copper-T) should be replaced, but the re-expulsion rate is about 50%.

5. *Perforation* (1 in 1000) occurs at the time of insertion. It is much more common following postpartum insertion when the uterus is soft.

There is usually a history of continuous pain from the time of insertion. The threads may be lost or still present.

The diagnosis is confirmed by ultrasound and abdominal X-rays. Copper IUCDs must be removed immediately by laparoscopy, or if necessary laparotomy, because they cause an intense peritoneal reaction and adhesions. The inert devices can be safely left in the abdominal cavity but they are best removed if it is easy to do so (i.e. laparoscopically).

The copper-T (Gyne-T) has the lowest perforation rate, 0:04 per 1000 insertions.

6. *Pregnancy*. There is a 2% failure rate per year. Most pregnancies occur with the IUCD *in situ* but pregnancy may follow perforation or expulsion. Once pregnancy is confirmed the IUCD should be removed, if the threads are still visible, whether or not the pregnancy is wanted. There is a high risk of ascending infection and the risk of abortion is about 50% whether the IUCD is removed or not.

If the threads have been drawn up, the IUCD must be recovered at delivery or termination and if it is not found then an abdominal X-ray is indicated to exclude perforation.

If the woman decides to keep the pregnancy, she can be reassured that there is no proven association between retained IUCD and congenital abnormalities.

1 in 20 pregnancies with an IUCD are ectopic (about 1 in 200 normal pregnancies); therefore if a period is late and there is abdominal pain, a laparoscopy may well be indicated.

The increased incidence of ectopics may be due to altered tubal motility or may be partly spurious because the IUCD cannot prevent ectopic pregnancy.

7. *Lost threads*. This may be due to:

— threads drawn up

— expulsion
— pregnancy
— perforation (rare)

a) Confirm by speculum that the threads are lost and examine to see if the uterus is enlarged (pregnancy).
b) If pregnancy can be excluded (e.g. within 10 days of period) use Spencer-Wells forceps or a Mi-Mark helix in the endocervical canal — the threads are often retrieved. If there is any chance the device has been displaced, remove it and replace another.
c) If the threads are not found, the cavity can be gently sounded (if pregnancy is impossible) and the IUCD may be identified. Otherwise an ultrasound scan will distinguish between the four possibilities and meanwhile the woman and her partner should use a sheath in case the device has been expelled.
d) If the IUCD is still in place, it can be left and scanned annually. Alternatively, the threads can be brought down by suction curette under local or curettage under GA.

IUCD removal

Gentle traction on the thread is usually all that is needed to remove the IUCD.

If this fails, it may be because the uterus is acutely anteverted or retroverted and applying a tentaculum to the cervix (after swabbing with antiseptic) and applying gentle traction may straighten the axis of the uterine cavity and allow removal.

If the threads break it may be possible to pass forceps into the canal and grasp the device.

The IUCD is best removed during a period or the first few days of the cycle if pregnancy is to be avoided (the contraceptive effect is reversed immediately). If pregnancy is planned it is usual to advise the woman to wait 1 month for the normal endometrium to regenerate.

The IUCD is left in for 12 months after the menopause and then removed, but any post-menopausal bleeding still merits a curettage.

N.B. Inert devices can be safely left, provided the woman has no symptoms and attends for annual smears. To change it exposes the woman to increased risk of pregnancy, perforation and infection. The devices are usually easy to remove, even after 15 years.

A Dalkon shield should, however, always be removed because of its association with pelvic actinomycosis.

The diaphragm

About 3% of married women in Britain use the diaphragm, but it is more popular in the United States, where women are more concerned about complications of the pill or IUCD

It has many *advantages*:

— effective: the failure rate is 2–3% per year but falls with age and with experience of the method

— no side-effects
— lowest mortality (including terminations for failures) other than vasectomy
— protection against carcinoma of the cervix
— spontaneity is not spoiled (unlike the sheath) because it is inserted beforehand and neither partner feels it during intercourse
— spermicide may help vaginal dryness

The *problems* with the method are that good motivation is necessary (it must be used every time), some women find the idea of inserting a diaphragm messy or unpleasant, a certain amount of dexterity is necessary (arthritis or weakness may make it impossible) and allergy to the spermicide can occasionally develop. Although they can be bought over the counter, they need to be fitted initially by a doctor or nurse. A diaphragm that is too large may cause mechanical urethritis and left in too long possibly predisposes to infection.

The diaphragm is a neat hemisphere of rubber with a flat metal spring in the rim. It works by holding spermicide near the cervix. A wide range of sizes are available but in practice the correct size will be a diameter of 65–85 mm (increasing in 5 mm steps except for 72.5 mm). The principle is to fit the largest diaphragm that is comfortable.

Fitting involves:

1. VE to examine the adnexae and cervix (screening) and to exclude cystocele, prolapse or poor vaginal tone which will prevent retention of a diaphragm. Retroversion of the uterus makes no difference (although fitting the diaphragm into the posterior fornix can be more difficult).

2. Assess the size needed by inserting the index finger into the posterior fornix and measuring the distance to the pubis.

3. A set of measuring rings can be used but a set of diaphragms is better. Choose a diaphragm of about the right size, the dome can be up or down (usually up) and compress the ring between finger and thumb.

Insert along the posterior vaginal wall until it is in the posterior fornix. The anterior rim is then pushed up behind the pubis.

4. The diaphragm fits diagonally across the vagina and covers the cervix and most of the anterior vaginal wall. If it does not cover the cervix, choose a larger size. If it causes discomfort choose a smaller size (it should not distend the vaginal walls).

5. Next the woman is taught how to insert the diaphragm, either squatting or with a foot on a chair. 'Compress the rim then push it downwards rather than upwards as far as possible, then push the anterior rim up behind the bone with your forefinger. Next check that the neck of the womb is covered by feeling it (like the tip of the nose) through the diaphragm.'

6. Demonstrate how to put cream on the diaphragm. A 10 cm strip is needed to inactivate an ejaculate and most of it should be put on the surface in contact with the os.

Provide the woman with a practice diaphragm of the correct size and see her in a week, with it in place (to have the position checked). During that week she should:

— practice inserting it with a spermicide
— practice wearing it during the day and during sex
— not rely on it for contraception

7. The following week, the position is checked and if the size is correct (no discomfort, not dislodged during sex or expelled by straining) a diaphragm of that size is prescribed.

Pain (backache, urethritis) means the diaphragm is too large and often the rim will be bent. Occasionally the diaphragm is too small and jams between the cervix and the pubis.

8. The diaphragm comes in a plastic box (like a powder compact). Spermicidal cream must be put on the diaphragm before insertion. A pessary is necessary if intercourse is delayed 2 hours or repeated; they take 5 minutes to melt.

The diaphragm can be bought over the counter but is free on prescription, e.g.

— flat spring Durex diaphragm 75 mm × 2
— duragel spermicidal cream 100 mg × 3
— orthofoam pessaries 15 × 3

The following points need to be explained (both verbally and with a leaflet if possible):

1. It must be used on every occasion and always with a spermicide.

2. It can be inserted at any convenient time before intercourse (the ideal would be routine insertion every night). If intercourse takes place over 2 hours after insertion insert additional spermicide (pessary or foam). If intercourse is repeated, insert additional spermicide.

3. Leave in place at least 6 hours after intercourse. On removal rinse in soap and water and dry. Do not leave in longer than 24 hours.

4. Walking about or urinating will not displace the diaphragm. A bowel movement may displace it, so check afterwards that it is still covering the cervix.

5. If a period starts with it in place, it does not matter, the blood will trickle around the edges. Leave it in for the full 6 hours and use a tampon as normal.

6. Inspect occasionally for holes and keep the rim circular. Do not stretch it and never boil it and it should last 2 years.

7. Have the size re-checked

— if weight changes by 10 lb (5 kg)
— 6 weeks postpartum (even a section)

— if vaginal surgery is performed
— every 12 months

Alternative barrier methods

1. *The vault cap* (Dumas) is a near hemisphere of firm rubber which covers the cervix and clings by suction to the vaginal vault. It is used when the vagina is too slack to retain a diaphragm. The size varies from 50 to 75 mm and the smallest size that maintains suction is used. It has to be inserted dome down but otherwise insertion and use are the same as the diaphragm. It is probably easier to dislodge than the diaphragm, especially on straining.

2. *The cervical cap* is thimble-shaped and varies from 22 to 31 mm in 3 mm steps, It is used when a diaphragm cannot be retained, but the cervix has to be long and healthy. It has a thread attached for easier removal.

3. *The Vimule cap* is a combination of a cervical cap and a vault cap, i.e. it is thimble-shaped with a wide flanged rim that also clings by suction to the vaginal vault. It can be used if there is a cystocele or a prolapse.

4. *The Vaginal Sponge* is a circular sponge, 5.5 cm, of polyurethane foam impregnated with the spermicide nonoxinol a (marketed under the name 'Today'). The sponge is moistened and inserted high in the vagina. It may be worn for 24 hours and should be kept in place for 6 hours after intercourse. It has a polyester loop to facilitate removal. It has several advantages over the diaphragm:

— one size suitable for most women
— no fitting required
— less messy
— additional spermicide not needed before each act of intercourse

There is still some concern that if left in the vagina there may be a risk of toxic shock syndrome. Some trials have found it to be as effective as the diaphragm, but most trials suggest it has a high failure rate and is best reserved for lactating women, those with reduced fertility (e.g. those over 45, or with secondary amenorrhoea) or those who want to become pregnant in a short period of time.

The Sheath

The 1544 Fallopius advocated the use of a linen sheath to protect against venereal disease.

Sheaths are also called condoms, Durex, protectives and French letters. The sheath is widely used and has several advantages:

— Highly reliable (used properly)
— No health risks
— Easily available
— Protective against venereal infections
— Possibly decreased carcinoma of the cervix

Used by well-informed and well-motivated couples, failure rates as low as 0.4 per 100 women years have been reported. Used incorrectly the failure rate is 20–30. The sheath has the disadvantage that it is coitus-related and therefore of low acceptability for some couples. Rubber allergy can develop. Sheaths are supplied in one size only.

Instructions for use
1. Use on every occasion
2. Use before any genital contact
3. Always use with spermicide
4. The man must hold it on when withdrawing
5. Use once only, before the expiry date

The sheath is not prescribable on FP10 but can be obtained free from Family Planning Clinics.

Spermicides   Spermicides can be used in conjunction with diaphragms, condoms, IUCDs or coitus interruptus to increase the effectiveness of contraception. They have a physical barrier effect as well as containing a chemical toxic to sperms (usually nonxinol 9). They should be inserted high in the vagina a few minutes before intercourse. There are various types:

— jellies (e.g. Duragel)
— creams (e.g. Orthocreme)
— pessaries (e.g. Orthoforms)
— foams (e.g. Emko foam)
— C — Film

Note: There is no evidence of increased risk of fetal abnormality in women who become pregnant while using spermicides.

Natural methods   Natural methods of family planning rely on abstinence during the fertile part of the cycle. This can be recognized by means of the calendar or by symptomothermal methods (or both).

These methods, especially in combination, can provide very effective contraception if used by well-motivated couples.

However, some couples practise withdrawal during the fertile phase of the cycle, making the method much less reliable.

1. The calendar method   The principle of the method is based on the fact that ovulation always occurs 14 days before a period. In a regular 28-day cycle the unsafe period has been found to be days 10–18. This is because:

— ovulation can vary around Day 14
— the ovum survives 1 day
— sperm in the female reproductive tract survives 3 days

Ideally the unsafe period should be stretched to allow for the longest and shortest cycles in the last 12 months: *If a cycle is short*, e.g. only 25 days, the follicular phase must be 3 days shorter than usual, so intercourse becomes unsafe 3 days earlier than usual, i.e. Days 7–18 instead of 10–18.

If a cycle is long, e.g. 32 days, the follicular phase is 4 days longer than usual, so intercourse remains unsafe for 4 extra days, i.e. Days 10–22 instead of 10–18.

N.B. The method is useless if periods are irregular, or the cycle-length varies by more than 10 days.

2. Symptomothermal methods

Ovulation can be detected by:

— temperature rise
— ovulatory cascade of mucus. The cervical secretions become watery and can be pulled out into a thread (spinbarkheit) the *Billings method*.

N.B. Intercourse should not occur until 3 days after ovulation has been detected by these methods.

Post-coital contraception

Reliable post-coital contraception is sometimes requested, or advisable (e.g. following rape). The DHSS has ruled that use of these methods within 72 hours of intercourse is legal and does not constitute an abortion.

Find out how long ago intercourse took place and make sure that unprotected intercourse has not also taken place earlier in the cycle. VE to exclude pregnancy.

The are two methods:

1. *The 'morning-after pill'*. Four tablets of Ovran or Eugynon 50 (pills containing 50 mg of ethinyloestradiol). Two pills as soon as possible and two 12 hours later. Given within 72 hours this is 99% effective. It is effective at any stage of the cycle. It is best to prescribe an anti-emetic as well.

50% get nausea. If vomiting occurs within 2 hours of taking the pills an IUCD should be considered.

A withdrawal bleed may occur a few days later and the next period may be delayed for a few days.

There have been no reports of thrombo-embolism following this method, although a history of such is probably a contraindication.

2. *The IUCD* is 100% effective up to 5 days afterwards, and has to be used if the woman presents after 72 hours or vomits the pills. It is also the method of choice if the woman is past day 18 of a 28 day cycle. It can be removed after the next period.

N.B. Discuss future contraception. Barrier methods are necessary for the rest of the cycle after the post-coital pills.

See the woman after her next period to make sure she is not pregnant and to discuss contraception.

Some doctors advocate providing a pack of four pills to couples using barrier methods, in case of accidents.

Sterilization Sterilization of one partner is a simple reliable method of contraception that is becoming increasingly popular. Sterilization of one partner is a simple reliable method of contraception that is becoming increasingly popular and is now the contraceptive method of choice for married or cohabiting couples (24% in 1983 compared to 4% in 1970). In 1983 roughly equal numbers of women and men were sterilized. It is ideal for the stable couple who are absolutely certain that whatever happens they will not want any more children and who have several years of potential fertility ahead of them (it may not be worthwhile if the woman is nearing the menopause).

Although it is expensive, it is cost-effective in community terms. A woman with an IUCD for 10 years has a theoretical 1 in 10 chance of an unwanted pregnancy followed by either termination (expensive) or childbirth which with increasing age is associated with increased PNM and maternal mortality.

Sterilization is essentially a destructive operation and counselling is important to avoid years of bitter regret. The GP is in the ideal position to be sure the couple are making a mature, informed decision and to advise his hospital colleague.

The couple should be seen together so they both clearly understand the procedure and its implications.

The following points need to be discussed:

1. Alternative methods
2. Irreversibility
3. Male or female
4. Female sterilization
5. Vasectomy
6. Side effects
7. Failure rate
8. Consent

1. *Alternative methods* will usually have been considered by the couple, but the GP should mention them (particularly POP, diaphragm, IUCD) and compare their merits or dismerits with sterilization. The advantages of sterilization should be discussed as well as the disadvantages.

2. *Irreversibility*. The procedure must be considered irreversible. Reversal is still only successful in 50%. In the female it requires complicated micro-surgery (time-consuming and expensive) and increases the risk of an ectopic by × 10. In the male reversibility is technically easy but only 50% achieve fertility, possibly because antisperm antibodies develop. Therefore the GP must enquire about factors which might make the request for reversal likely:

— both young (or one partner much older)
— recent or sudden decision
— psychiatric history
— stability of marriage (sexual, social, financial)

— number and ages of children (? under one year)
— medical condition of children

3. *Male or female?* The couple will usually have already decided but may ask the doctor for advice:
It should obviously be performed on the woman if she has health reasons to avoid future pregnancies. History or examination may reveal indications for a hysterectomy.

— fibroids
— menorrhagia
— abnormal smear
— prolapse
— ovarian mass

If for one partner it symbolizes genital trauma (despite reassurance) it is best avoided.

Vasectomy is quicker but takes 3 months to have contraceptive effect. The risks of failure or complications (haemorrhage, infection) are equal; (Vasectomy is also easier to reverse and has a lower mortality of 1 in 100 000 compared to 10 per 100 000).

4. *Female sterilization*
This can be achieved by:

— laparoscopy (clips, rings, diathermy)
— laparotomy (Pomeroy or Irving technique)
— hysterectomy
— vaginal approaches (culdoscopy, colpotomy)

Laparoscopic sterilization using Hulka-Clemens *clips* (plastic with a metal spring) is usually the method of choice. The fibre-optic laparoscope is introduced via a 1 cm incision in the lower umbilical fold and the clip applicator is inserted through a separate incision. It is a difficult operation technically, but only a small area of tube is damaged, causing less postoperative pain and good potential for reversibility. Some surgeons put two clips on each side to decrease the failure rate (about 1 in 500). The Filshie clip is being increasingly used. It is made of titanium and lined with silicone rubber which expands as the fallopian tube necroses. It is simple to apply.

The woman is advised to stop the pill for a month before (thrombosis) and use a sheath. The procedure is timed to avoid her luteal phase (in case she is already pregnant) and she and her partner should use a sheath until her next period. It is usually performed under GA; she is allowed home when she is free of pain, usually the next day, and is off work about a week.

— *Rings* cause more postoperative pain from the strangulated loop of tube (1 in 500 fail)
— *Diathermy* is irreversible (4 cm of tube destroyed) and gut can get damaged (1 in 500 fail)

— *Laporotomy* and tubal ligation via a suprapubic incision is necessary if the woman is very obese or has pelvic adhesions. Post-abortal sterilization should be avoided for emotional reasons. It can be performed after elective caesarian section or within 72 hours of delivery (via an incision at the level of the fundus) if the woman made the decision early in pregnancy.

The original *Pomeroy* ligation has a 1 in 500 failure rate (up in 1 in 50 on vascular postpartum tubes). The *Irving* technique (proximal stump is buried in the myometrium) has a failure rate of 1 in 1000.

Excised tube should be sent for histology (to prove it is fallopian tube).

— *Culdoscopy* or *colpotomy* are rarely performed
— Insertion of tubal plugs via a transcervical hysteroscope remains experimental.

5. *Vasectomy* is a simple safe outpatient procedure performed under local anaesthetic, and takes about 20 minutes. Bilateral short incisions are made high in the scrotum, each vas is dissected free, 2 cm excised and the ends doubled back to prevent recanalization.

A GA may be necessary if there is a varicocele or hydrocele. (Ligation of the vas can also be performed during a herniorraphy or prostatectomy).

Postoperatively an athletic support should be worn day and night for a week, to avoid pain. Scrotal bruising is often dramatic but usually subsides in a few weeks without treatment. The risk of a haematoma is decreased by 2 days off work with no heavy lifting. Occasional complications are:

— haematoma (3%; icepacks; drain if large)
— infection (antibiotics)
— epididymo-orchitis (rarely)

The volume of ejaculate is unchanged. Sperm clearance takes about 20 ejaculations. Negative counts at 12 and 14 weeks is considered safe. Persistent sperm occurs rarely due to operative error or double vas, and this requires re-exploration. The failure rate (1–3 per 1000) is due to recanalization.

Vasectomy is cheaper than female sterilization, (requiring less expertise, equipment and time both to perform and reverse).

6. *The mortality* of female sterilization, which involves opening the peritoneum, is about 1 in 10 000, and mortality is virtually nil for male sterilization (1 in 100 000). *Complications* of infection or haemorrhage arise occasionally with equal frequency.

Many people fear effects on their masculinity or femininity, libido, sexual performance, volume of ejaculate, etc., and explanation with diagrams of the mechanical nature of the procedure is important. A common question is what happens to the egg/sperm (which are absorbed by normal body processes).

Some women complain of heavier periods and should be warned of this if they will be stopping the pill. In most others it is probably coincidental dysfunctional bleeding and there is no evidence that sterilization has any endocrine effects. Long term follow-up of vasectomy patients has revealed an increase in anti-sperm antibodies but no harmful systemic effects in man.

7. The couple must be aware that sterilization can fail (1–3 per 1000), due to recanalization or poor operative technique. After tubal occlusion about 20% of such pregnancies are ectopic.

8. *Written informed consent* must be obtained from the person being sterilized, who must be over 16. The consent of the partner is not legally necessary but must always be obtained where possible. If the decision is not unanimous, sterilization should normally be postponed because it can worsen a poor relationship (one partner can have risk-free extramarital intercourse).

A mentally-handicapped person cannot be sterilized because they are not legally capable of giving valid consent.

In summary:

1. Counsel both partners (together if possible) about family, irreversibility, method and effects and failure rate (diagrams are useful to stress the mechanical nature of the operation)

2. Examine the woman vaginally (to exclude indications for hysterectomy)

3. Consent from both partners.

Termination   Therapeutic abortion is legal if there is a risk (greater than if the pregnancy was terminated) to:

1. the woman's life (0.3%, e.g. heart, renal, carcinoma)
2. the physical or mental health of the woman, or
3. her family, or
4. risk of a handicapped child (Rubella, Down's syndrome, neural tube defect)

These conditions of the 1967 Abortion Act are listed on the 'green form' (Form HSA1) which must be signed by two doctors. Parental consent is needed if the girl is under 16.

The actual wording on the form is: 'We hereby certify that we are of the opinion, formed in good faith, that in the case of .... (name and address of patient)

1. the continuance of the pregnancy would involve risk to the life of the pregnant woman greater than if the pregnancy were terminated;

2. the continuance of the pregnancy would involve risk of injury to the physical or mental health of the pregnant woman greater than if the pregnancy were terminated;

3. the continuance of the pregnancy would involve risk of injury to the physical or mental health of the existing child(ren)

of the family of the pregnant woman greater than if the pregnancy were terminated;

4. there is substantial risk that if the child were born it would suffer from such physical or mental abnormalities as to be seriously handicapped.

Clause 1 allows any abortion to be deemed legal since it can be interpreted to mean that any termination under 12 weeks is statistically safer than a full-term pregnancy.

The need will persist for the forseeable future but could be decreased if more attention were paid to the *possible causes*:

1. Contraceptives never used — probably 50%. Improved education and availability would decrease these.

2. Failed contraception — either bad luck (rare), incorrect usage or deliberate sabotage by the partner

3. Lapsed contraception:

— carelessness (often the beginning or end relationships)
— subconscious reason (e.g. to punish self or boyfriend or parent, to provide an alternative love object, or disgust at having to be premeditative about sex)

Education about contraception and counselling to uncover subconscious motives offer the best hopes to decrease the number of requests. Repeat abortions account for only 9% of abortions performed.

The doctor may reasonably adopt one of the following attitudes to termination:

1. Never (a doctor is legally allowed to opt out)
2. To save the woman's life
3. For the woman's social well-being
4. On demand

Social well-being is part of the WHO's 1949 definition of health, but is variously interpreted by doctors, who tend to project their own social framework onto the patient. A situation included by one doctor would be excluded by another. Because of this, many doctors offer termination on demand (under part 2 of the 1967 Act). 80% of patients have made a firm decision on presentation. 20% need counselling, when the role of the doctor is to lead the patient to make her own decision, remembering that a few women will want the doctor to say 'no'. The doctor should point out the option of continuing the pregnancy and having the baby adopted.

Termination in the first trimester is a safe procedure with a mortality of only 1 per 100 000. Mortality rises steeply with gestation:

Weeks	Mortality rate per 100 000
16	15
21	35

Complications also rise with gestation, and 5% will get serious complications after 16 weeks.

— perforation
— haemorrhage
— infection
— cervical tears

There is an *increased incidence* of subsequent:

— ectopics
— infertility
— cervical incompetence
— premature labour

The earlier the termination, the less the risk. After 14 weeks dilatation of the cervix becomes necessary to remove all the fetus and the risk of morbidity or mortality rise steeply due to:

— cervical damage
— retained products (haemorrhage, infection)

Late abortions are sometimes indicated for:

— fetal abnormality (amniocentesis)
— maternal illness (hypertension, renal, carcinoma)

1. *Under 6 weeks.* This is euphemistically called 'menstrual regulation' and is more commonly practised in the USA than in Britain. If the period is late by 14 days or less, the uterus is evacuated using a 4–6 mm flexible Karman cannula and a 50 cc gynaecological syringe to provide the vacuum. It can be performed with or without paracervical lignocaine (which decrease cramping afterpains). A pregnancy test need not be awaited.

2. *Under 14 weeks.* Vacuum aspiration using a size 12 Karman curette under GA. This is the safest method, and is best performed at 8–10 weeks (earlier than this, and the small sac can be missed).

3. *After 14 weeks* there are two possible methods:

a. Dilatation and surgical evacuation using ovum forceps to break up the fetus. Prostin in tylose can be inserted into the posterior fornix 24 hours beforehand to soften the cervix and so decrease the trauma of dilating it up.
b. Extra-amniotic prostaglandin infusion. A Foley catheter is inserted through the cervix and an infusion of prostaglandin (5 mg of prostaglandin E_2 (Prostin) in 50 ml of saline at 1–2 ml per hour) is started i.v. Syntocinon can be given as well. An epidural is often used, because the contractions are very painful. Abortion takes about 24 hours and can be an emotionally unpleasant experience.

Retained products are common, and surgical evacuation under GA is usually needed.

Other techniques have a much higher complication rate and are rarely used now:

— hysterotomy
— intra-amniotic instillations (saline, urea, prostaglandin)

In summary:

1. Perform VE to confirm gestation. Vacuum aspiration if less than 14 weeks.

2. Check blood group. If Rhesus negative, give 50 mg of Anti-D.

3. Discuss contraception. Start the pill Day 1 after the abortion or insert IUCD.

4. Prevent infection. Antibiotics can be given either for prophylaxis (especially for late abortions) or at the first sign of infection (discharge or fever).

5. Follow-up has shown that few women suffer psychological effects. About 5% still feel guilty at 8 weeks, especially after late abortions. A major cause seems to be hostile staff attitudes.

Research in contraception   1. *Barrier methods.* Research into a more acceptable material than latex rubber is in progress. Improved packaging, labelling and counselling services could improve efficacy.

The *non-spermicide fit-free diaphragm* is a 60 mm diaphragm that can be worn continuously.

2. *The IUCD* is often associated with pain, bleeding or expulsion. The Progestasert device, which releases 65 μg per day of progesterone, causes less problems but needs changing every year.

Biodegradable microspheres are likely to be available for contraception soon. They are placed in the vagina, migrate through the cervix and release a steady concentration of progesterone over several years.

3. *Suppression of ovulation.* Constant low dose hormone delivery by *subdermal sialastic implants* (needing surgical insertion and removal) or vaginal rings (possible hygiene problems). New analogues of oestrogen and progesterone may allow lower doses to be used in the pill.

Analogues of LHRH given daily (as nasal spray) paradoxically suppress ovulation and have a half-life of under 5 minutes and few toxic effects. Long-acting analogues are, a possibility.

4. *Vaccines* to induce antibodies to HCG (killing the blastocyst) and, even better, to the zona pellucida (preventing sperm penetration) are being developed. Experimentally the contraceptive effect is reversible. An anti-FSH vaccine for men would depress spermatogenesis without affecting testosterone secretion.

5. *Tubal sclerosants* would allow outpatient sterilization. The problem is one of delivery to the tubes. A device for injecting

methylcyanoacrylate (a fast-setting glue) has been developed.

An IUCD has been developed with quinacrine (a sclerosant) on the tips of the transverse arms.

6. *Detection of ovulation* Computerized thermometers and kits to detect urinary hormone changes are being developed. Kits to predict ovulation would greatly increase the effectiveness of natural methods.

7. Advances in micro surgical techniques make reversible *sterilization* an increasing possibility.

8. Early abortion (*'menses induction'*) and using analogues of prostaglandin and anti-progesterone may become available for monthly use or when the period is late by a few days.

Breast examination Many carcinomas still present as large lumps, and teaching *self-examination* of the breast is probably a useful method of screening. The following is one method of teaching.

1. The best time routinely to feel for lumps is after a period, lumpiness (fibroadenosis) is commonly felt.

2. Look at the breasts in the mirror, then raise the arms, looking for assymetry or nipple inversion.

3. Use the flat of the hand and four fingers to feel for lumps (the finger-tips can detect the normal lumpiness of the glandular issue).

4. Feel all the breast (with the opposite hand) systematically ('like the face of a clock'), pressing the breast against the ribs. Explain how the axillary tail of the breast tissue extends into the armpit and should not be missed.

A mammogram is simply a low intensity soft tissue X-ray that uses the inherent contrast of breast-tissue to show pathological changes. They are easier to interpret after the menopause (increased fat with fibrosis of glandular tissue). A rounded benign lump can often be distinguished from an irregular carcinoma but nevertheless biopsy is always indicated.

It can detect lumps of only 0.5 cm that are still impalpable and may be useful for screening especially in

— strong family history
— previous carcinoma (6% are bilateral)

Breast lumps 1. Fibroadenoma
2. Fibroadenosis
3. Cyst
4. Carcinoma

1. *Fibroadenoma* (age 20–30) is a lump that is characteristically very mobile (the breast mouse). The girl is usually in her 20s. It is treated by excision biopsy — 'no woman should have a lump in the breast'.

2. *Fibroadenosis* (age 20–50) is due to multiple small cysts (epitheliosis blocking the ducts) usually in the upper outer

quadrant. It is uncomfortable and tender and worse before a period and settles down again once the period is established. It tends to be worse when periods are irregular and there may be other features of pre-menstrual tension (fluid retention, headache, irritability). It is cured during a pregnancy. Management involves:

— Reassurance and see in 2 weeks when it will have settled.
— Mild analgesies and a firm bra. Frusemide 40 mg daily for the 4 days before a period often helps. Alternatively bromocryptine or danazol are both effective.
— If further reassurance is needed, aspiration of one of the larger cysts or mammography (multiple rounded lesions of variable density) can be helpful.

3. *A cyst* (age 40–50) usually appears suddenly, often just before a period and most commonly in the last 5 years before the menopause. It may be in an area of fibroadenosis (the pathology is the same). Treatment is by aspiration and biopsy is unnecessary, provided:

— the lump disappears completely
— the fluid is not uniformly blood stained
— the fluid is negative on cytology
— the cyst does not rapidly reform (see in 1 month)

Cysts never occur a year after the menopause.

4. *Carcinoma* of the breast (age 40–80). Over the age of 60 a lump will be a carcinoma (unless there is a clear history of recent severe bruising, when it may be fat necrosis). The lump is single, hard, irregular and non-tender and there may be tethering or nipple inversion or discharge, skin nodules or palpable nodes.

Prognosis depends on whether metastases are already present (25% even of early lesions) and not on the method of removing the primary. Simple lumpectomy followed by radiotherapy produces as good a survival rate as any other method.

Venereal infections
— syphilis
— gonorrhoea
— NSU
— genital herpes
— genital warts
— molluscum contagiosum
— tropical (chancroid, LGV)

Pubic lice, scabies, *Candida* and trichomoniasis can also be spread venereally.

Hepatitis B, *Giardia*, *Shigella* and amoebiasis are probably transmissable by the venereal route.

There are *two important principles* in the management of all venereal diseases.

1. If one venereal infection is present, always exclude the others.

2. Trace and treat all contacts, a difficult task best performed by specially trained nurses or social workers.

AIDS   Acquired Immune Deficiency Syndrome (AIDS) is a lethal syndrome characterized by unexplained opportunistic infections and aggressive Kaposi's sarcoma. First reported in May 1981, affecting particularly homosexual men in New York and San Francisco, the incidence of AIDS has increased exponentially, doubling every six months. The doubling time in Britain is currently about 10 months. There have now been 600 cases reported in Britain and 20 000 in the United States (January 1987) There are 50–100 times this number of sero-positive persons.

The spectrum of HIV disease   Once antibody tests were developed it became clear that there is a spectrum of HIV disease. Antibodies are produced 4–8 weeks after exposure. 10% of sero-positives will develop AIDS after an incubation of 1–3 years (see Fig. 2).

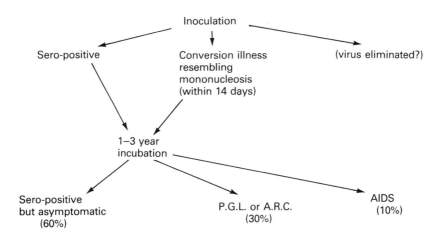

Fig. 2

The Conversion Illness lasts 3–14 days, with fever, headaches, arthralgia, macular rash, sore throat and generalized lymphadenopathy. Sero-conversion occurs 3–8 weeks later.

Progressive Generalised Lymphadenopathy (PGL) consists of unexplained lymphadenopathy in at least two extra-inguinal sites (especially axilla and posterior cervical) for more than three months. There is little constitutional upset. 90% are sero-positive. The prognosis is good and only 20% will progress to AIDS over a 3 year period. Lymph node biopsy shows only follicular hyperplasia and excludes non-Hodgkins lymphoma (found in 5% of AIDS patients). Constitutional symptoms (fever, weight loss, malaise, chronic diarrhoea) indicate a progression to *AIDS-related complex* (ARC).

ARC is defined as two or more symptoms or signs (hepato-splenomegaly, oral infection) with two or more abnormal lab tests (leucopenia, anaemia, raised ESR, thrombocytopenia, raised immunoglobulins). A high percentage will develop AIDS.

AIDS   *AIDS is defined as*:

1. The presence of a reliably diagnosed disease indicative of cellular immune deficiency.
2. The absence of a recognizable cause for immune deficiency (e.g. transplant patient).

The patient will be sero-positive.
The diseases indicative of cellular immune deficiency are:

Malignancies (histologically proven):

— Kaposi's sarcoma under the age of 60.
— B-Cell lymphoma
— Primary lymphoma of the brain.

Opportunistic infections (with lab confirmation):

— Pneumocystis pneumonia
— Toxoplasmosis (lung, CNS)
— Cryptococcus (meningitis or disseminated)
— Candida (oesophageal, lung)
— Salmonella spp
— Atypical mycobacteria
— Campylobacter
— Herpes simplex (mucocutaneous ulcers for more than 1 month)
— CMV (re-activation)
— Progressive multi-focal leukoencephalopathy (papova virus)

(Other infections occur but are very uncommon in the U.K. e.g. Cryptosporidium, Cryptococcus, Histoplasmosis, Aspergillus, Microsporidium, Nocardia, Actinomycetes and Legionella.)

N.B. Serology is unreliable because of poor antibody response. Diagnosis depends on isolation of organisms or histology.

Risk groups

	% of cases UK	USA
Homo or bisexual	89	73
IV drug abusers	1	17
Association with Africa	3	—
Recipients of blood products	5.5	3
Heterosexual contacts	1	1
Unknown	0.5	6

Passive anal intercourse and sexual promiscuity produce the greatest risk. Heterosexual transmission does occur. Being Haitian is not a risk factor, Haitian cases have now been associated with other risk factors. The disease originated in central Africa and was carried to Haiti by immigrant workers. It is a new disease in man probably spread from an animal reservoir. Antibodies to HIV have been detected in stored serum from central Africa from 1972. AIDS has been reported in woman who have had *artificial insemination* of infected donor sperm. All *donor blood* is now screened for antibodies and factor VIII is heat-treated, so the risk to haemophiliacs is now greatly reduced. Heterosexual transmission is more common in Africa although the picture is confused by the use of unsterilized needles, the use of anal intercourse as a means of contraception and mosquitoes and other possible vectors.

Virology

The epidemiological similarities to hepatitis B led to the search for a virus, identified in 1983 at the Institute Pasteur in a patient with PGL and called lymphadenopathy associated virus (*LAV*). A year later the virus was isolated by the Institutes of Health in Bethesda, USA, from a patient with AIDS and called Human T-cell lymphotropic Virus (*HTLV-III*). The virus is now called the *Human Immunodeficiency Virus (HIV)*.

It is a retrovirus with single-stranded RNA characterized by a unique enzyme, *reverse transcriptase*, which synthesises virus-specific double-stranded DNA which is integrated into the cell chromosome and acts as a template for viral RNA (therefore it is a persistent virus and once caught it is carried for ever — like Hepatitis B, Herpes simplex, Herpes Zoster and CMV). Two retroviruses HTLV-I and HTLV-II have already been linked with acute and chronic T-cell leukaemia of adults.

The virus has now been isolated from most body fluids but *blood* and *semen* are the main vectors of transmission. The virus shows marked tropism for T-helper cells, using the T4 cell surface antigen as a receptor. The virus also infects monocytes and neural cells. Loss of helper T-cells has a devastating effect on the immune system because they orchestrate both T and B-cell activity. Antibodies to envelop antigens appear weeks or months after infection but only low levels of neutralizing antibody develop, therefore blood of sero-positive individuals remains potentially infectious. An effective *vaccine* is unlikely because antibodies are non-neutralizing and because the virus shows antigenic variation. *Antiviral agents* are being developed such as reverse transcriptase inhibitors (e.g. azidodeoxythymidine or AZT).

Testing for HIV infection

Detection of the viral antigens involves cultivation of lymphocytes and an assay for reverse transcriptase or hybridization assays to detect viral RNA in brain tissue. The virus is isolated in a continuous T-cell line only for research purposes.

The presence of antibody implies continued infection (because the virus persists in host cells) but occasionally carriers of the virus do not develop antibodies. Rapid, sensitive and specific tests for antibody detection are available but no one test is ideal and the laboratory will need clinical details to determine which tests are appropriate.

HIV carriers

Carriers are asymptomatic and identified by routine screening. It is estimated there are 100 times more carriers than cases. In London 35% of homosexuals are sero-positive, and 80% of severe haemophiliacs. Their main problems are psychological.

Counselling sero-positive patients

Confirming the presence of HIV antibodies is a dreadful pronouncement. One patient wrote an article on the subject entitled 'Don't tell me on a Friday', because immediate and detailed counselling is needed. The information is a shock and the person needs to express fears, discuss uncertainties and come to terms with the changes in life-style. The main points are:

— The sero-positive person does not have AIDS. They are *infectious* to others and have a 20% chance of developing AIDS, but most will remain healthy. Explain facts and prognosis.
— Infection is spread sexually and in blood (urine and saliva may also be infectious). Avoidance of transmission involves safe sexual practices, i.e. mutual masturbation and 'dry' kissing and current advice is against both vaginal or anal sex (both may be safer with a condom).
— Dentists and surgeons must be warned of the dangers. The person must not donate blood, organs or sperm. Advise against ear-piercing and tatooing. Toothbrushes should not be shared. Touching, kissing and using the same toilet are not risks.
— Reassurance about confidentiality as far as possible.
— Contact tracing, where this is relevant.

N.B. The Terrence Higgins Trust have a help-line with trained counsellors. Telephone 01-242 1010.

Clinical aspects of AIDS

The clinical picture can include:

— Weight loss, fever, lymphadenopathy
— Dry cough (pneumocystis)
— Persistent oral thrush
— Purple skin lesions (Kaposi's)
— Diarrhoea (Salmonella, CMV, Cryptospordium)
— Peri-anal ulceration (Herpes simplex)
— Headaches (Cerebral abscess)
— Progressive dementia (HTLV-III encephalopathy)
— Cachexia and death

50% present with *Pneumocystis*, with dry cough and fever but often no signs and a normal CXR initially. There is hypoxia and a marked reduction in carbon monoxide transfer. Bronchoscopy is essential for diagnosis (midzone brushings). Asthma tends to worsen. Treatment is with high-dose Septrin 8 tabs b.d. 80% get a macular-papular rash on Septrin, which is not an indication to stop treatment but if the rash involves mucosae the treatment is changed to Pentamidine. Candida pneumonitis and atypical TB also occur.

Oral Thrush can be extremely difficult to eradicate, and commonly involves the oesophagus. Long-term Ketoconazole (Nizoral) is needed. Leukoplakia also occurs in the mouth and can be mistaken for thrush.

Kaposi's Sarcoma is a vascular neoplasm previously seen as an indolent condition in elderly males. Kaposi's plaques typically appear first on the palate. Purple skin lesions resembling bruises enlarge into nodules. Gut involvement occurs. The prognosis is better with Kaposi's alone, without opportunistic infections. There is also an increased incidence of B-cell lymphoma.

Diarrhoea is a common problem due to salmonella, CMV (that can cause toxic dilatation of the colon) and cryptosporidium. Cryptosporidiosis causes profuse watery diarrhoea (like cholera) and is diagnosed by a Ziehl-Neelsen stain. It is rapidly fatal. There were only twelve cases in the world literature before 1982. There is often an associated bacteraemia (e.g.: Salmonellosis) which is difficult to eradicate with antibiotics.

Peri-anal ulceration and induration occurs due to chronic herpes simplex infection. It responds well to Acyclovir. Squamous carcinoma of the anal margin is more common (possibly associated with wart virus).

20% present *with CNS symptoms*. Encephalitis can occur due to CMV, Herpes simplex or cryptococcus. CT Scan is indicated to exclude a cerebral abscess (toxoplasmosis or candida) and lumbar puncture may be indicated. Brain biopsy worsens prognosis.

CMV Retinitis can cause bilateral blindness. Cotton wool spots on the retina are highly suggestive of impending opportunistic infection.

Cerebral atrophy and dementia can occur, thought to be due to invasion with HTLV-III virus itself. *Dementia* is a possibility even in those successfully treated for opportunistic infections.

Death occurs 1–2 years after diagnosis. Survival depends on presenting disease (see below). Infections become more frequent and more difficult to eradicate. Weight loss and wasting occur even in the absence of infections. In addition to infections a presenile dementia can occur due to primary brain infection with HIV virus.

Prognosis   *Mean survival from first diagnosis*

Kaposi's alone	125 weeks
Pneumocystis alone	35 weeks
Other opportunistic infections	18 weeks

Nursing the AIDS patient   The AIDS patient does not need to be nursed in isolation. Percutaneous inoculation is the only risk of transmission. Goggles and masks are unnecessary. The virus is very delicate and sputum, vomit, urine and faeces are not infectious. The virus is inactivated by mild disinfectant (e.g.: Miltons). Salmonella diarrhoea or TB (atypical mycobacteria) are indications for isolation, and the patient should be nursed in a side-room if bleeding or incontinent. The risk of infection to health workers is very low. Only one out of 73 staff known to have suffered needle stick injuries with needles used by AIDS patients became sero-positive after 3 years (compared to 35% following Hepatitis-B needle injuries).

Inactivation of the virus   The decontamination procedures for hepatitis B are more than adequate for HIV since it is a more labile virus. 10% household bleach is suitable for disinfection of spilled blood. Equipment such as endoscopes should be soaked in 20% activated glutaraldehyde for 15 minutes.

AIDS and pregnancy   Sero-positive women should be advised against pregnancy or to postpone the decision until more knowledge is available. A woman with a sero-positive partner should not become pregnant, because the risk of AIDS is increased in pregnancy.

If a seropositive woman becomes pregnant, termination should be advised because there is a 50% risk of transplacental transmission to the baby and a 50% risk of AIDS in the sero-positive baby.

The prognosis for both mother and baby is poor. Pregnancy seems to increase the risk of progression to AIDS. AIDS develops within two years in 50% of babies (average age 7 months) with failure to thrive, oral thrush, pulmonary infiltrates, pneumocystis and Herpes simplex.

Syphilis   There were 4000 case, of syphilis in the UK in 1981. It is caused by the spirocheate *Treponema pallidum* which can invade intact mucosa or enter via an abrasion, e.g. the finger. The four stages are:

1. *The primary chancre* develops about 3 weeks (9–90 days) after contact, usually on the vulva or penis (or anus in homosexuals, ressembling a fissure).

A pink papule breaks into an ulcer which is painless, rounded and oozes serum. Untreated, it heals in 3–8 weeks. The inguinal nodes are usually enlarged, but are rubbery and non-tender.

Diagnosis involves dark ground illumination of the serum for spirochaetes; repeat daily for 3 days. Serology does not become positive until around 6 weeks — repeat monthly for 3 months. Keep the ulcer clean with saline but never give antibiotics until the diagnosis is certain. Follow up for 2 years.

2. *Secondary syphilis* develops about 6 weeks after the chancre appeared, with fever, myalgia, malaise and:

— rash (non-itchy, symmetrical, maculo-papular lesions involving palms and soles; sometimes alopecia) — 75%
— Generalized lymphadenopathy (rubbery and non-tender and including epitrochlear and suboccipital nodes) — 50%
— Mucosal ulcers (snail track) — 10%, or perineal 'warts' (condylomata lata) — 10%. Both team with spirochaetes if dark ground illumination is used on the serum.

Untreated these manifestation resolve over a period of months and the patient passes into the stage of *latent syphilis* with positive serology but no other involvement, including aortic (CXR) and CSF (lumbar puncture). Even without treatment 60% have no further progression.

3. *Tertiary syphilis* is rarely seen nowadays. It occurs 3–10 years after primary infection and is characterized by gummas (granulomas) mainly of skin, mucosa and bone (but rarely viscera) that heal with penicillin.

4. *Cardiovascular or neurological complications* develop in about 10% of untreated cases after 5–30 years. They are due to endarteritis and fibrotic damage to the aortic ring, causing:

— aortic incompetence
— angina
— aortic aneurysm (ascending and calcified)

and damage to meninges and nerve roots, causing:

— Meningovascular syphilis (headache, cranial nerve palsies, root pain)
— Tabes dorsalis (dorsal column degeneration)
— GPI (cortical degeneration and dementia)

Serology   The modern screen for syphilis is the VDRL (introduced 1946) together with the TPHA (introduced 1967). Both are cheap and simple.

1. *The VDRL* detects an antibody (reagin) which for some reason is present in high titre in syphilis and causes clumping of lipoidal antigens (flocculation).

It is positive in 75% of primary syphilis and is ideal for follow-up because it becomes negative with treatment.

False positives occur in:

— viral illness, vaccinations
— glandular fever
— SLE
— rheumatoid arthritis

2. *The TPHA* detects specific anti-treponemal antibodies

that haemagglutinate sheep red cells. False positives are less likely.

If only one test is positive repeat the screen; if both tests are positive perform an FTA.

3. *The FTA* (introduced 1964) was devised to overcome the problem of false positives. It labels the treponemes with specific fluorescent antibodies. It is the most sensitive test and is highly specific. It is the first to become positive (at 6 weeks) and remains positive for life. It is time-consuming and expensive.

Management

1. In pregnancy all women are screened at booking and if 'at risk' the tests are repeated at 35 weeks.

2. Syphilis confirmed by FTA is treated with procaine penicillin 600 000 units i.m. daily for 10 days, or benzathine penicillin, 2.4 Mμ weekly for 2 weeks. In penicillin allergy oral erythromycin for 2 weeks is effective.

Inadequate treatment means that the patient is susceptible to the late complications. Treatment even late in pregnancy usually leads to the birth of a healthy child.

3. Untreated syphilis in pregnancy tends to cause abortion or stillbirth. Later pregnancies in a syphilitic woman can to term and the child may have *congenital syphilis* (bloodborne, therefore no primary stage), with:

— rash and lymphadenopathy
— bloodstained nasal discharge (osteo-chondritis)
— gummas and neurosyphilis (late)

Diagnosis in a baby is proved by the IgM–FTA test, although this may not be positive until 9 weeks. It is treated with penicillin.

Gonorrhoea

Gonorrhoea is now the most prevalent infectious disease in the world apart from the common cold, due to increasing promiscuity among the young and the development of drug resistant gonococci. There were 58 000 cases in the UK in 1981.

Neisseria gonorrhoeae is a Gram-negative intra-cellular diplococcus that invades tissue not covered with stratified squamous epithelium (urethra, cervix, Bartholin's glands).

In men, it causes dysuria and urethral discharge 2–5 days after contact. In women, it is often symptomless, but dysuria, frequency and vaginal discharge may occur after about 2 weeks. Trichomoniasis co-exists in 60%. It can persist as a chronic and contagious disease for years and is the commonest cause for blocked tubes.

Complications

— salpingitis, bartholinitis (epididymitis)
— proctitis, pharyngitis (anal or oral sex)
— vulvo-vaginitis (children)
— bacteraemia (fever, rash, septic arthritis)
— neonatal opthalmitis (blinding)

Gonorrhoea must always be suspected in acute salpingitis, especially if there has been no recent delivery or abortion and the woman does not have an IUCD.

The best method of *diagnosis* is to take charcoal swabs from the urethra and cervix and transport in Stuart's medium for plating within the hour. In men, a Gram stain of discharge is 95% accurate, but in women commensal organisms complicate the picture and culture is necessary.

The *treatment* is one oral dose of 2 gm ampicillin plus 1 g probenecid. Eight tablets of co-trimaxazole is effective if the patient is allergic to penicillin. Follow-up is essential, because resistant organisms are becoming common. Repeat the swabs at 2 weeks and, if gonococci are isolated, spectinomycin 4 gm i.m. is indicated (expensive). Syphilis must always be excluded.

Nonspecific urethritis (NSU)

There were 130 000 cases of NSU in the UK in 1981. Men develop dysuria and mucoid urethral discharge, usually 2–3 weeks after contact. It is probably due to *Chlamydia* but most clinics make the diagnosis on a Gram stain of discharge, showing pus cells but no gonococci. Complications are prostatitis, epididymitis and Reiter's syndrome (5%). It is treated with a 3-week course of tetracyclines, during which intercourse is best avoided. It tends to recur and can be very difficult to eradicate.

The female partner should also be treated (with erythromycin if pregnant) as there is evidence that relapse in the man is then less likely once intercourse is resumed. Chlamydial infection in the female is usually symptomless but can cause:

— salpingitis
— cervicitis and infertility
— chlamydial conjunctivitis in the newborn

Genital herpes

This is the commonest cause of vulvo-vaginal ulceration in Britain. There were 12 000 cases in the UK in 1981. It is due to *Herpesvirus hominis* (HVH) type II. It is transmitted sexually, and 4–5 days after contact, a burning sensation develops, then a cluster of tiny vesicles which soon rupture, leaving painful erosions usually on the vulva but sometimes on the cervix.

The primary infection is often severe, with fever and malaise, root involvement (pain, difficulty micturating) and painful inguinal lymphadenopathy or iliac fossa pain (the cervix drains to the iliac nodes). Rarely, meningitis or hepatitis is seen.

Cervical herpes usually causes severe necrotic ulceration, but the virus can be shed from a normal-looking cervix. The recurrent attacks are less severe and are usually precipitated by sexual intercourse.

The clustering of vescicles is very distinctive, but syphilis must always be excluded in any genital ulceration. Definitive diagnosis is by swabs and cervical scrapings for viral culture (which produces characteristic cell changes). Paired sera will show a rising titre after a primary attack.

Treatment
— The ulcers will heal in 10 days as long as secondary infection is prevented. Potassium permanganate baths are soothing and povidone iodine helps prevent secondary infection.
— Analgesics are needed if root pain develops. Urinary hesitancy always resolves and catheterization should be avoided if possible.
— If secondary infection occurs; use Septrin, which does not mask syphilis. Check serology at 3 months to exclude syphilis.
— Genital herpes in the last month of pregnancy is an indication for elective section (neonatal encephalitis can occur).
— Acyclovir is a potent and specific antiviral agent which is active against Herpes simplex types I and II. The pain and other symptoms of the primary infection are reduced by acyclovir (oral or IV), but subsequent recurrence rate is not reduced. Acyclovir cream only reduces the severity of the recurrent episodes if applied early (before vesicles appear). Continuous use has been shown to suppress recurrent attacks, but when treatment stops recurrences return. It has no serious side-effects.

Genital warts
Condylomata accuminata are caused by a papova virus and transmitted sexually. There were 34 000 cases in the UK in 1981. The incubation period is around 3 months (1–6 months) and they occur in an older age group than skin warts. They occur on the vulva and perineum, but may extend up the vagina.

In moist areas, they become large and filiform and in immunosuppressed patients can become very large. They are unsightly, cause itching, irritation and discharge and they may bleed. In a few patients, treatment is ineffective but like hand warts, they eventually disappear.

Management
1. Topical podophyllin (10–25%) in spirit or in tincture of benzoin. It is applied weekly to the warts and washed off 6 hours later. It is very irritant to normal skin, which should be protected during application with Vaseline. If skin irritation occurs 2% hydrocortisone cream is useful. Some podophyllin gets absorbed and it is teratogenetic and therefore must never be used in pregnancy. The consort should be treated if warts are present or should use a sheath to prevent infection.
2. Multiple warts are best treated by diathermy under general anaesthetic.
3. Exclude other venereal infections. Trichomoniasis commonly co-exists.

Molluscum contagiosum causes painless, fleshy papules that are easily recognized because of a central umbilification, out of which cheesy material can be squeezed. They are caused by a very large DNA poxvirus. They spread by direct contact and can occur on any part of the body. Podophyllin is effective. There were 1000 cases in the UK in 1981.

Tropical veneral infections
— Chancroid
— L.G.V.
— Granuloma inguinale

1. *Chancroid* can mimic primary syphilis. It is a disease of the promiscuous and unhygienic and is largely confined to seaports of the Far East, Africa and South America. In 1981 there were 100 cases reported in the UK.

It is due to *Haemophilus ducreyi* which is extremely difficult to culture. 2 or 3 days after contact, painful ulcers develop on the genitals. Inguinal nodes become tender and enlarge and can develop into an abscess. Diagnosis usually has to be clinical but syphilis (usually a single painless ulcer with rubbery non-tender nodes) must be excluded by dark ground illumination. The treatment of choice is co-trimoxazole, which also has the advantage that it does not mask syphilis.

2. *Lymphogranuloma venereum* (LGV) is a venereal infection due to a Group A chlamydia that is confined to tropical seaports. There were 41 cases in the UK in 1981. About 3 weeks after contact, small painless ulcers develop which usually go unnoticed in women, then chronic inguinal lymphadenitis, with sinus formation and caseous discharge, usually with fever and weight loss.

If untreated, labial perforation develop, and fibrotic scarring with fistulae, rectal and urethral strictures and lymphoedema. Epitheliomas can develop in the involved skin.

It is diagnosed by a complement fixation test (better than the Intradermal Frei test), and co-trimoxazole is the treatment of choice.

3. *Granuloma inguinale* is an uncommon chronic skin condition virtually confined to coloured races in tropical regions. There were 29 cases in the UK in 1981. It is of low contagiousness and is thought to be spread venereally.

About 7 weeks after contact, painless ulcerating granulomas develop in the perineal region, eventually healing with fibrosis. Biopsy stained with Giemsa demonstrates the diagnostic Donovan bodies in monocytes, described in 1905 and now thought to be bacteria of the *Klebsiella* group. Tetracyclines produce healing.

Psychosexual counselling
The incidence of sexual problems is unknown. Surveys reveal that 15% of men and 30% of women feel they have sexual problems of some kind. Referral rate for counselling is only about 6 cases per 10 000 population (i.e. 1–2 cases per GP) per year. There are three landmarks in the development of our present attitudes to sex.

1. In 1949 Kinsey published statistical reports showing that sexual activity (both homo- and heterosexual) was much more widespread than had generally been assumed, and he saw sex as a powerful innate force that demanded expression.

Sex is of course extremely important to all of us, and many people view the loss of sexual function as more important than losing an eye or a limb.

2. In 1966 Masters and Johnson published *Human Sexual Response*. Using volunteers in a laboratory setting, they analysed the physical events of sexual intercourse and demonstrated that women also have orgasms and that they are always due to clitoral stimulation. They developed a therapy to treat sexual problems, but concentrated on the physical rather than the emotional aspects of sex.

Ignorance about the plain facts of the anatomy and physiology of sexual intercourse still causes many psychosexual problems.

3. In 1974 Alex Comfort published *The Joy of Sex* and emphasised that sex should be recreational and not just a battle to achieve as many orgasms as possible. He pointed out that sex has a therapeutic and relaxing effect that drains away aggression.

Inherent in this view of sex as an enjoyable game is the assumption that both partners have communicated about the rules. Social myths about what each partner should feel and do, together with lack of communication about what each partner would like to do, are the commonest causes of psycho-sexual problems.

Counselling is a form of psychotherapy. All this means is that lasting change is achieved by listening and talking. To be effective, only 2 things are required of the therapist:

a) The right sort of personality. A therapist can rarely help someone he does not like. He has to feel empathy and respect (even respect for bizarre fantasies) and he must form a relationship with the person or couple, who will not abandon beliefs or attitudes at the behest of an uncaring stranger.

b) He must be willing to interact and express his own feelings.
Given that the therapist is sensitive and has healthy atti-tudes to sex, his own true feelings about the subject are the best way to lead the patient to a useful new understanding and awareness. This demands pesonal honesty from the therapist, who must also have no preconceived ideas about the likely areas of conflict causing the problem. The Masters and Johnson method involves giving the couple tasks to do at home, then counselling on emotional reactions and communication.

In practice many psychosexual problems can be resolved by simple discussion and common sense.

No two people are the same. To help a couple with a sexual problem, a doctor must understand his own attitudes, be willing to listen sympathetically and be able to offer a working voca-bulary, e.g. 'do you have problems with lack of sexual appetite, poor lubrication, having a climax, ejaculating too soon, keeping an erection' etc. Depending on the problem, a very detailed history is usually necessary. The following is merely a check list:

Psychosexual history

1. *The problem*. It usually falls into one of the following categories:

— libido
— stimulation
— intercourse
— orgasm

2. *Intercourse*. Has it ever been enjoyable? Frequency, pain or difficulty (impotence, premature ejaculation, vaginismus). Frequency of orgasm. Contraception.

3. *Periods*. (Does she use tampons or towels?) Any infertility. Obstetric history is very important (e.g. termination, stillbirths, pueperal frigidity, attitudes to breast-feeding)

4. *Sexual history*. Attitudes, derived from family and education. Fantasies or recurring dreams. Masturbation. Previous sexual experiences (heterosexual, homosexual, incest, rape).

5. *Personal history*. Friends, relationships, school, career, achievement, religious and moral attitudes. Marital or extra-marital relationships.

6. *Social history*. (Family, housing, job.)

7. *Past medical*, drug or psychiatric history.

The GP is often the ideal person to help a couple with sexual problems. Patients often disguise the problem, sometimes for years, and the possibility of psychosexual problems should be considered in patients with multiple symptoms (the 'thick file syndrome').

Many psychosexual problems are solved using simple common sense to improve communications. However, not every couple can be helped. Some simply no longer have any love for each other, some are in a neurotic collusion that defies solution, some have deep-seated personality problems.

Counselling can be time-consuming. Patients can be referred to trained psychosexual counsellors via a Family Planning Clinic or Marriage Guidance Council.

The problems are categorized here into:

1. Physical causes
2. The relationship
3. Ignorance
4. Social myths
5. Fear of failure
6. Failure

1. Physical causes

These are usually obvious, but nevertheless must not be overlooked. *Superficial dyspareunia* may be due to candidiasis, trichomoniasis or atrophic changes. Sometimes an episiotomy scar or congenital abnormality requires plastic surgery.

Deep dyspareunia may be due to endometriosis or chronic salpingitis and may be an indication for laparoscopy. Sometimes chronic cervicitis causes deep pain and requires cryocautery.

Premature ejaculation can rarely be due to urinary infection, prostatitis or neurological disease.

Impotence is usually psychological but consider:

— depression
— alcohol
— drugs (hypotensives, thiazides, anxiolytics, steroids, cimetidine)
— diabetes neuropathy (50% over age 60)
— pituitary tumour (either causing hyperprolactaemia or hypopituitarism with low FSH and LH *serum testosterone* will be low in both cases)

An intra-cavernosal injection of an α-blocking drug e.g. phenoxybenzamine can be self-administered and causes an erection for several hours.

Loss of libido can be due to general ill-health e.g. hypothyroidism, chronic renal failure (improves with dialysis) or psychiatric illness, e.g. schizophrenia.

2. The relationship

Sexual problems often dissolve once the relationship between the couple improves. Conversely, sexual problems cannot be solved while a relationship remains poor.

The problem is nearly always one of *poor communications*. Conflicts about children, relatives, job etc. may be unresolved. One partner may be suffering low self-esteem, either mental (depression), physical (obesity, post-natal, post-menopausal, coronary, colostomy, mastectomy, hysterectomy) or social (unemployment, isolation).

The doctor can offer guidelines for re-establishing communication, e.g. setting time aside for discussion and openly stating emotional feelings. The doctor often somehow acts as a catalyst, and simply discussing the problems with the couple may be all that is needed.

3. Ignorance

Ignorance about the basic anatomy and physiology involved is still common. Before explaining anything find out what is not known.

Foreplay and mutual stimulation are often hampered by attitudes like 'men automatically know what to do' or 'women should be passive' or 'it's wrong to talk during sex'. The doctor can encourage sexual communication by suggesting leading the partner's hand to touch sensitive areas and telling each other what they feel like.

There may be ignorance about the need for both clitoral and vaginal stimulation and for female lubrication. There may be strange fantasies about what the vagina is like inside (e.g. 'like tissue paper') which may be dispelled by a vaginal examination and explanation (ideally with the partner present) and by teaching the woman to examine herself.

Only the doctor can examine someone physically, and he should never waste the opportunity of saying 'everything is normal'.

4. Social myths   Social myths still abound and most of them are variants of the following:

— 'Nice woman don't do it'
— 'Real men don't show their feelings'

Inappropriate feelings, originating from parental, school or religious attitudes have often been retained. The doctor, as a similar figure of authority is in a good position to reverse these and to 'give permission' for more healthy feelings and to 'give permission' for masturbation, oral sex or whatever the couple enjoy doing together. Merely discussing sexual matters openly is a form of permission giving.

5. Fear of failure   This always develops when there is sexual tension. Once the above problems have been resolved, anxiety about performance can be reduced by redefining 'success' simply as shared pleasure. If both partners are enjoying the experience, it does not matter how aroused each partner becomes relative to the other.

A simple way to reduce performance pressure is to ban intercourse for a while and have regular sessions of mutual carressing when demands for intercourse are not made — the 'sensate focus' technique of Masters and Johnson. The couple should be encouraged to say what they are not enjoying, so the partner knows that what they are doing is enjoyable for the other.

6. Failure   Temporary failure of intercourse may be due to tiredness, prying children or a creaking bed! More permanent problems are:

— premature ejaculation
— impotence
— vaginismus
— poor lubrication
— anorgasmia

Premature ejaculation is due to loss of voluntary control over ejaculation. Usually the man is trying to take his mind off the feelings in the mistaken belief that this will help prolong intercourse. He has to be taught to concentrate on recognising the pre-ejaculatory sensation. The best method of overcoming the problem is 'the squeeze technique'. He signals to the woman just before ejaculation and she pinches the glans for about 30 seconds until the sensation goes away. As he gets better at control he will learn to stop every so often during intercourse.

Impotence is usually psychological (guilt, low self-esteem, marital conflict) and this is confirmed if the man can have erections at other times, e.g. early morning, by masturbation or with other women. Simple counselling often relieves the problem.

Vaginismus is often due to unreasonable guilt feelings or fears of pain or damage based on ignorance or fantasies and can often be relieved by patient explanation, examination and teaching self-examination. Graded dilators for use at home are often helpful. Sometimes it is due to deep-seated rejection of adult status and then requires prolonged psychotherapy.

Poor lubrication is usually due to inadequate stimulation by the man, but KY jelly is sometimes useful. Exclude atrophic vaginitis.

Some women enjoy sex without ever achieving orgasm. The man may feel inadequate because he cannot 'give' the woman an orgasm. Often it is because she is not sufficiently relaxed to 'let herself go' completely.

Obstetrics

Maternal death is defined internationally as the death of a woman while pregnant or within 42 days of termination of the pregnancy (irrespective of site or duration). Causes are sub-divided into:

— Direct (Pregnancy complication or management)
— Indirect (Previous disease aggravated by pregnancy)
— Fortuitous (e.g. accidents)

Maternal mortality has fallen from 500 per 100 000 total births in the last century (due to haemorrhage, sepsis, pulmonary embolus and disproportion — rickets) to 99 in 1951 to 8. 9 per 100 000 in 1981. Maternal deaths now form less than 1% of all deaths of women in this age group (compared to 4% in 1952–54).

The confidential enquiry also looks separately at *late deaths* (43 days to 1 year) after delivery or abortion. In 1979–81 there were 66 late deaths and 5 were considered direct (2 choriocarcinoma, 1 post partum cardiomyopathy, 1 pulmonary embolus, 1 sepsis post LSCS).

Since 1952 a 3-yearly report called the *Confidential Enquiry into Maternal Deaths in England and Wales* has analysed maternal deaths and particularly emphasised avoidable factors.

Maternal mortality has fallen substantially. In the tenth and latest report (for 1979–81) there were 176 *direct maternal deaths* (the figures for the previous 3 reports being 340, 227 and 217) or 72 deaths per million pregnancies (the figures for the previous 3 reports being 124, 96, 95). The fall is probably due to improved maternity services and maternal health, due to:

— better social conditions
— improved health
— antibiotics, transfusions, safe surgery
— falling parity
— confidential enquiries, and hence
— improved maternity services
— more hospital deliveries

In the event of a maternal death the area Medical Officer initiates an enquiry. An enquiry form (MCW97) is sent to the G.P., midwife, consultant and any other staff involved in the woman's case. These are sent to the CMO and a team of assessors who review all the available recorded facts about each case. Patients are not named and all the forms are later destroyed.

Causes

Causes of direct Maternal mortality (1979–81)	Number of Deaths	
Hypertensive disease of pregnancy	36	(20.4%)
Pulmonary embolus	23	(13.0)
Anaesthesia	22	(12.5)
Ectopic pregnancy (excluding anaesthetic deaths)	20	(11.4)
Amniotic fluid embolus	18	(10.2)
Haemorrhage	14	(8.0)
Abortion (excluding anaesthetic deaths)	14	(8.0)
Sepsis (excluding abortion)	8	(4.6)
Ruptured uterus	4	(2.2)
Other direct causes	17	(9.7)
	176	(100%)

The report stresses the following points:

1. Maternal mortality from *hypertensive disease of pregnancy* (PET and eclampsia) has not changed significantly since 1970 (47 cases). It was considered that management was substandard in 27 out of the 36 deaths (95%). Causes of death were cerebral haemorrhage or oedema (failure to control hypertension), hepato-renal failure (inadequate monitoring of liver function and DIC) and post-partum cardiac failure due to fluid overload (the vascular bed is reduced in severe PET and fluid balance needs expert control).

The aim of expert care is to deliver the infant before complications threaten the life of mother or fetus. The aspect of care where improvements are needed were:

— Routine antenatal care (earlier detection)
— Control of Hypertension
— Prevention of Fits
— Anticipation of Liver damage
— Anticipation of DIC
— Timing of delivery and fetal monitoring
— Intravenous fluid overload (3 deaths)

Since severe PET is rare, the report recommended the formation of regional centres with special expertise to advise or take over difficult cases, and offer pre-pregnancy counselling and post-partum follow-up.

2. Deaths from *Pulmonary embolus* were the lowest since the reports started (23 plus 5 following abortion), but are likely to remain a significant cause of maternal death until significant advances occur in detection and prevention. 7 deaths occurred within 42 days of caesarian section. It is difficult to diagnose DVT during pregnancy and a high index of suspicion is needed, especially where there are risk factors: age over 35, high parity, obesity, prolonged antenatal bedrest or LSCS. A combination

of risk factors or a past history of DVT or PE may be indications for prophylaxis (subcutaneous heparin e.g. 5000 units t.d.s.). DVT should be confirmed by venogram and promptly treated with i.v. heparin. Oestrogens are no longer given to suppress lactation.

3. There were 22 deaths due to *anaesthetic complications*. 8 died from aspiration of gastric contents, 6 cardiac arrest, 6 cerebral anoxia, 1 respiratory arrest, 1 pulmonary oedema. The report stresses that cricoid pressure must be applied correctly with the neck fully extended otherwise intubation becomes difficult. Pethidine causes gastric stasis and a N/G tube and gastric aspiration should be considered. Cyanosis can be missed especially in dark-skinned patients and careful observations (pulse, BP especially) are needed for at least 30 minutes after the anaesthetic. Severe kyphoscoliosis is a very high anaesthetic risk.

4. *Ectopic pregnancy* deaths at 20 have not increased in number (21 in 1976–78) but have become a major cause of death as other causes have fallen. Death can occur even before any menstrual disturbance, and an acute abdomen or sudden collapse in any woman of child-bearing age may be an ectopic (NB even if the woman has been sterilized, has an IUCD in situ or in on any type of oral contraceptive). Laparotomy is indicated if the patient is shocked. In doubtful cases beta-H.C.G. (produced by the trophoblast 7 days after conception) ultrasound or laparoscopy will help to increase the accuracy of diagnosis.

5. *Amniotic fluid embolus*. No causative factor has been identified. The main danger is making the diagnosis too readily, and missing treatable causes of shock, e.g. ruptured uterus, DIC, septic shock.

6. *Haemorrhage*. In 9 out of the 14 cases care was felt to be substandard. 5 were APH (3 placenta praevia, 2 abruption) and 9 immediate PPH. Self-neglect by the patient contributed to 3 deaths. The report emphasises that each unit should have an agreed policy for the management of catastrophic haemorrhage. The risk from placenta praevia increases dramatically with the number of previous caesarian sections (because the placenta adheres to the scar). Blood transfusion needs careful monitoring and CVP control to avoid under — and over — transfusion. Coagulation failure must be suspected and detected early and managed in conjunction with a haematologist. Where PPH is more likely (high parity, previous twins) the woman must be delivered in a hospital i.v. infusion for the delivery and group and save serum). A woman with a retained placenta at home needs a flying squad.

7. *Abortion*. 14 deaths (7 sepsis, 5 PE, 2 haemorrhage). There were 5 deaths following legal abortion and in none was care considered substandard. Since the Abortion Act was introduced in 1968 the total number of deaths from abortion has

declined dramatically. The safest method of *termination* is by vacuum aspiration and the earlier the safer. The risk rises sharply after 12 weeks.

8. *Sepsis.* 8 deaths (4 postoperative, 2 puerperal, 2 infection of the amniotic cavity). Another 7 deaths due to infection post-abortion. Despite the wide range of antibiotics available death from sepsis still occurs. The delay of preterm labour with rito-drine can be particularly hazardous. If infection is suspected every effort must be made to isolate organisms from the genital tract and blood cultures and early discussion with microbiologists is essential.

9. *Ruptured uterus.* Care was regarded as substandard in 3 out of the 4 cases, and included the use of oxytocic drugs in 2 multiparous women. Treating a multip with oxytocics is hazardous, especially for intrauterine death because higher doses may be used without the risk of fetal distress. Uterine rupture should always be considered as a cause of shock, particularly in a multip on oxytocics.

10. *Other causes.* (14 deaths). 6 unknown, 5 due to fatty liver of pregnancy, 1 liver disease, 1 purulent mastitis, 1 massive haemoptysis on i.v. heparin.

There were 16 deaths from *cardiac disease*, 3 direct (3 cardio-myopathies), 9 indirect (3 congenital, 4 infarcts) and 4 fortuitous.

There were 92 *indirect maternal deaths* from pre-existing disease aggravated by pregnancy and the report stresses the 5 deaths from respiratory failure in women with severe *kyphoscoliosis.*

Caesarian sections were performed more frequently and there were 87 deaths (80 in 1976–78). One third of all direct deaths occurred in women delivered by caesarian. The death rate from emergency section (80 per 100 000) is much higher than for elective section (20 per 100 000).

Perinatal mortality (PNM)   PNM is defined as the number of stillbirths, plus deaths in the first week, per 1000 total deliveries. It is used as the measure of obstetric competence, although the ideal index would include the incidence of perinatal morbidity.

PNM has steadily fallen from around 500 per 1000 in deprived areas during the 1850s to 35 per 1000 in 1958 to 18 per 1000 in 1979 to 11 per 1000 in 1986. The PNM is lower in several other countries, e.g. Sweden, Holland. About 50% are neonatal deaths, mostly in LBW babies.

The fall in PNM is due to:

— improved health of the population
— reduced parity
— the surveys themselves, hence
— better maternity services
— screening for fetal abnormalities
— better neonatal care

The causes are:

1. *Congenital abnormalities* (either stillbirth or neonatal death). The main ones are anencephaly, hydrocephaly, spina bifida and gross cardiac lesions.

2. *Stillbirths* due to intra-uterine anoxia (i.e. placenta failure). Diabetes and rhesus disease cause a small number.

3. *Prematurity* mostly by causing RDS or due to gross immaturity (under 1 kg) $\mp$ infection

4. *Birth anoxia* $\pm$ trauma

How can PNM be reduced? Considering each of the causes in turn:

1. Geographic variation in the incidence of congenital abnormalities suggests that there are causes to be found and perhaps removed (see section on Preconception Clinics for discussion of vitamin supplements pre-conception). Avoid drugs in early pregnancy. Check the rubella state of women before pregnancy if possible and vaccinate if necessary. Amniocentesis can detect neural tube defects. Some abnormalities e.g. duodenal atresia can be detected prenatally by scan and corrected promptly by surgery.

2. Know the risk factors and select the high risk patients for delivery in a unit with monitoring facilities and an SCBU. Detect gestational diabetes by knowing the indications for a GTT. Diagnose PET early by good antenatal supervision. Admit for monitoring if placenta failure is likely (IUGR, PET, Diabetes, APH, postmaturity, previous small infant).

3. Decrease the incidence of premature labour where possible. Suture for cervical incompetence. Decrease the number of early inductions by good management of PET and diabetes and be certain of gestation (i.e. early booking) especially before social inductions. Possibly bedrest for twins or a previous history of premature labour. Ritodrine can often stop premature contractions. Dexamethasone given to the mother for 48 hours before delivery may decrease the chance of RDS. Move immediately to a unit with an SCBU if premature labour starts.

4. Active management to prevent long labours (hypoxia, infection) and intrapartum monitoring to detect fetal hypoxia which predisposes to cerebral haemorrhage. Remember that forceps and section increase the risk. Facilities for immediate resuscitation and intensive care in an SCBU are the most important factors.

The high-risk case   'High risk' means there is a statistically increased chance of PNM or perinatal morbidity. High risk cases should ideally be booked for delivery in consultant units with facilities for intrapartum monitoring, 24 hours anaesthetic cover and attached SCBU. Antenatal management decisions (e.g. where to book for delivery, when to admit for monitoring, when to induce labour) are based on a knowledge of *which factors are associated with an increased PNM. These are*:

1. Maternal factors
   — age over 35
   — parity (first or fourth +)
   — low SEC
   — heavy smoking
   — height under 5 feet (152 cm)

2. Bad past obstetric history
   — abortion, ectopics
   — APH, abruption
   — premature labour
   — LSCS
   — fetal abnormalities
   — perinatal deaths

3. Present complications
   — diabetes, hypertension
   — APH
   — rhesus antibodies
   — IUGR
   — severe anaemia
   — twins or hydramnios
   — premature labour
   — malpresentaion
   — postmaturity

Antenatal care is based on a knowledge of these risk factors.

However, 50% of perinatal deaths have no identifiable risk factors at booking. 50% of patients selected as suitable for confinement without specialist attention develop complications (antenatally or in labour) necessitating a change of plan. Therefore the type of antenatal care

— specialist
— shared care
— community

and the place of birth may need to be changed if risk factors develop.

Preconception clinics   1. To further reduce fetal malformation, a better understanding of early pregnancy is necessary, e.g. vitamin supplementation around the time of conception might possibly reduce neural tube defects (NTD). There is evidence that vitamin supplements taken for a month before and three months after conception reduces the recurrence rates of NTD from 4.2% (about 1 in 25) to 0.5% (1 in 200).

The incidence of anencephaly was shown to be seasonal in 1951 (Record and McKeown) and minor vitamin deficiencies in winter were suspected as a cause. Women carrying NTD fetuses were shown to have slightly reduced vitamin levels. This prompted Smithell's work.

His trial (Smithells R.W. et al, Lancet, 7 May 1983, p1029) used a combination of folate and vitamins (Pregnavite Forte F). It was not randomized but compared women (all with a history of NTD) who accepted vitamins (2 NTD recurrences in 406 mothers) to those who either refused or were already pregnant — the controls (19 NTD recurrences in 468 mothers). This striking reduction suggests that folate plus vitamins may well reduce the risk of recurrence and should be given to all women with a history of NTD who wish to conceive.

Since 95% of NTD pregnancies have no past history (and since pregnancy is not usually confirmed until after neural tube closure at 28 days) it can be argued that all women should have vitamin supplements when stopping contraception. The MRC trial of folate versus placebo may answer this question (although results may be difficult to interpret because the incidence of NTDs is anyway falling). Meanwhile the importance of a good diet prior to conception has been emphasised, although there is no evidence that the recent vogue for measuring the trace element content of hair is of any value at all in assessing nutritional status.

2. The woman with worries because of recurrent abortions or previous stillbirths, abnormal babies or a family history of abnormality can seek expert opinion and genetic counselling. Tests for carrier status of a specific abnormal gene may be requested (e.g. for sickle cell anaemia. Tay-Sachs disease or β-thalassaemia). Couples needing detailed counselling should be referred to a geneticist, who can assess recurrence risks accurately (e.g. retinitis pigmentosa can be inherited as an autosomal dominant, autosomal recessive or X-linked disorder.) Screening techniques and the possibility of therapeutic abortion can be discussed.

3. Women with chronic medical conditions can be advised about pregnancy. Diabetic control can be optimized by glycosylated Hb (HbA_{ic}) levels and fetal abnormalities possibly reduced. Renal and cardiac problems can be assessed before pregnancy and drug regimen (anticonvulsants, anticoagulants, steroids) modified.

4. Routine antenatal care can be further improved.

— date of LMP certain
— rubella status checked
— exclude anaemia, syphilis
— avoid drugs
— check pre-pregnancy BP
— stop smoking and avoid alcohol
— early booking (so gestation is accurately known)

Heavy smoking in pregnancy results in a reduced birth weight of 150–200 g (placental vasoconstriction and fetal carboxyhaemoglobin causing fetal hypoxia and growth retardation). It also causes a 20% increase in abortion and 20% increase in neonatal death rate.

Heavy drinking at any stage of pregnancy can cause the fetal alcohol syndrome (growth retardation, dysmorphic features, mental retardation) and even moderate drinking (2 drinks per day) can cause minor abnormalities.

5. This is the ideal time for the couple to start considering the options and to think about how they want to have their baby (see the section 'Alternative Methods of Childbirth').

Diagnosis of pregnancy   Gestation in weeks is given in brackets.

1. The *symptoms* of pregnancy are:

— missed period (4)
— nausea (4)
— tiredness (6)
— breast tingling (6)
— urinary frequency (6)
— fetal movements (16–18)
— colostrum, tightenings (20)

2. The *signs* are:

— cervical softening (6)
— nipples pigment (8)
— enlarged uterus
— large egg (8)
— orange (10)
— uterus palpable above pubis (12)
— fetal heart heard (24)
— fetal parts felt (28)

3. *Tests*:

— Urine test. The proprietary kits (Gravindex, Pregnosticon) detect urinary HCG 11 days after a missed period (in a 28 cycle), but false positives and negatives can occur. They become negative at 20 weeks.
— Ultrasound scan can detect the gestation sac at 6 weeks and the fetal heart at 7 weeks.
— Doppler (e.g. Sonicaid) can detect the fetal heart at 12 weeks.

Early development   1. The blastocyst implants 7 days after fertilization. It consists of an outer trophoblast layer (the future chorion), an inner cell mass and between them a chorionic space. It becomes buried beneath the decidua by the action of the trophoblastic enzymes.

2. The inner cell-mass forms an embryonic plate (the future fetus) and an amniotic cavity which expands *to surround the fetus*, except for the cord, and obliterates the chorionic space (like a balloon expanding in a balloon); hence the membranes consist of 2 layers (outer chorion and inner amnion).

3. As it grows, the conceptus forms a bump beneath the decidua which enlarge to fill the whole uterus by 12 weeks.

The decidua overlying the conceptus fuses with that on the opposite side (hence salpingitis, i.e. ascending infection, cannot occur after 12 weeks of pregnancy because the tubes are 'blocked off').

4. The part of the trophoblast that first implanted becomes the placenta and develops villi. The placenta can be identified by scan from 12 weeks and after this time an abortion is a mini-labour rather than expulsion of the conceptus as one clot.

5. The umbilical vessels (2 arteries, 1 vein) end as capillaries in each villus; thus the fetal circulation is closed. The spiral arteries of the uterus spurt maternal blood into the intervillous spaces, hence placental bleeds consist of maternal blood.

6. By 8 weeks organogenesis is complete and the fetus is a miniature human the size of a jelly baby.

Physiology of pregnancy   1. The placenta produces:

— HCG
— oestriol, progesterone
— HPL
— prolactin

Prolactin and HPL cause breast development. The corpus luteum also produces relaxin which probably causes softening of the cervix.

2. *Progesterone* levels are high in pregnancy, produced in the first 10 weeks by the corpus luteum (supported by HCG from the trophoblast) and later by the placenta.

Levels fall during the last 5 weeks of pregnancy (possibly increasing uterine contractility). The actions of the progesterone are:

— Glandular development (decidua, breasts)
— Decreased myometrial activity
— Decreased smooth muscle tone of:
  a) stomach and colon (possibly to slow gut motility and increase absorption but predisposing to heartburn and constipation)
  b) ureters (dilated until 12 weeks postpartum and predisposing to pyelonephritis)
  c) Veins (predisposing to varicose veins — together with the pelvic 'tumour' effect — and helping to lower the diastolic BP by 10–20 mmHg — together with the low resistance circuit of the chorio-decidual space of the placenta)
— Progesterone is responsible for the dyspnoea of pregnancy, causing chronic hyperventilation and lowered maternal P_{CO_2} (hence easier transfer of fetal CO_2).

3. *Oestriol* is the predominant oestrogen and is synthesized by the 'feto-placental' unit via:

— maternal pregnanolone (from cholesterol)

— fetal adrenal (converted to de-hydro-epiandrosterone)
— fetal liver (hydroxylated)
— placenta (hydrolysed oestriol)

Oestriol causes uterine growth (the uterus increases from 60 g to 1000 g) and softening of ligaments of the pubic symphysis (increasing pelvic size), and lumbar spine (allowing a lordosis to carry the fetus but predisposing to root pain) and ribs (splaying to allow room for the fundus).

Oestriol is not essential for pregnancy. In the very rare placental sulphatase deficiency, oestriol is absent yet pregnancy is normal.

4. *Sodium retention*, due to raised cortisol and aldosterone levels with:

— increased blood volume — about 30% by 30 weeks
— increased cardiac output — about 30% by 12 weeks
— haemodilution
— oedema (carpal tunnel syndrome)

Cortisol causes gluconeogenesis but insulin levels are also raised so blood glucose levels are normal. Glycosuria is common because the renal threshold is lowered.

5. *Weight gain* of pregnancy is about 10 kg (0.5 kg per week) for the last 20 weeks). This is due to:

— fat and fluid — 5 kg
— fetus — 3.5 kg
— placenta — 1 kg
— amniotic fluid — 0.5 kg

Metabolic rate is increased in pregnancy and goitre can occur, but the free thyroxine index is normal.

6. *Lab values* changed:

— increased red cell mass
— lower Hb (e.g. 11 g/dl — haemodilution. MCH and MCV normal)
— raised WBC (up to $16 \times 10^9/1$ — mainly neutrophils)
— raised platelets (as high as 600 000 in the puerperium)
— raised ESR 30–100 (increased globulins)
— raised fibrinogen and clotting factors (vii, viii, x)
— plasma viscosity remains normal
— decreased albumen
— increased alkaline phosphatase (placental)
— increased cholesterol
— increased creatinine clearance (raised cardiac output and glomerular filtration, e.g. 200 ml/min)

The obstetric history

1. *Name, age, parity* (e.g. 2 + 2, the second figure refers to abortions)
2. *LMP* (? normal, or in fact a threatened abortion)
3. *Was pregnancy planned* (? infertility, ? pill)

4. *Gestation* (by dates and early scan); gestation at booking

5. *Past obstetric history* (obstetric problems tend to recur):

— any abortions (cervical damage)
— dates of deliveries (or ages of children), and details of each:
— antenatal (diabetes, PET, APH)
— labour (? premature, induced, prolonged)
— delivery (? forceps, section, PPH)
— baby (? alive, birth weight, condition at birth, breast fed)

6. *Details of this pregnancy*:

— serial weight, BP, urine
— scans or amniocentesis
— fetal movements (from 16–18 weeks)
— minor symptoms
— admissions (vomiting, bleeds, diabetes, PET, growth retardation)

7. *Past medical history*

— drugs or allergies
— uterine scars, vaginal repairs, cervical surgery, ectopics
— pelvic fractures
— blood transfusions, general surgery
— illness (cardiac, respiratory, renal, neurological, haematological, psychiatric)

8. *Family history* (diabetes, hypertension, Down's syndrome, spina bifida, anencephaly)

9. *Social history* (husbands occupation; smoking)

10. *Height, shoe size* (under 5 feet = 152 cm, makes disproportion more likely)

The antenatal routine   *Booking* (ideally at about 10 weeks):

— full obstetric history
— breasts (? nipples inverted)
— chest and heart (? mitral stenosis)
— uterine size
— VE (smear, cyst or fibroids, discharge)
— urinalysis, blood tests
— scan to confirm gestation
— discussion (importance of antenatal visits, value of oral iron, general advice)

Subsequent antenatal visits should occur:

— monthly to 28 weeks (at 28–30 weeks, ? small for dates)
— fortnightly to 36 weeks (at 36 weeks, ? breech)
— weekly to term (refer at term + 10 days)

At each visit the routine is:

— gestation? (by dates and early scan)

— symptoms? fetal movements?
— weight, BP, urinalysis
— uterine size (? agrees with dates)
— presentation, position, fetal heart

Notes   1. *Blood* is taken at booking for:

— Hb, group (sickle test, Hb electrophoresis and stools for parasites should be considered in immigrants)
— VDRL
— antibodies (rhesus, rubella)
— serum alphafetoprotein (15–20 weeks)

Blood is taken again at 28 and 36 weeks for:

— Hb
— antibodies (if rhesus negative)

Positive VDRL is usually a false positive due to a recent viral illness or previous infection with yaws (in immigrants), and FTA will then be negative.

If the woman has no rubella antibodies she should be immunized in the puerperium.

A high serum *alphafetoprotein* is an indication for amniocentesis. It is performed at 16 weeks. Only 1 in 20 of those with high serum levels will have an abnormal fetus. It is high in anencephaly, spina bifida, exomphalos, impending fetal death and twins.

2. *Fundal height* is approximately:

symphysis — 12 weeks
(halfway — 18 weeks)
umbilicus — 24 weeks
(halfway — 30 weeks)
xyphisternum — 36 weeks

The uterine volume and fetal size are also assessed by palpation from about 28 weeks.

3. *Small-for-dates* (admit for full fetal monitoring):

— wrong dates (e.g. early amenorrhoea was due to stopping the pill).
— fetal abnormality (Potter's syndrome, chromosomal abnormalities)
— placental insufficiency

4. *Large-for-dates* (scan):

— wrong dates (LMP was in fact a threatened abortion)
— twins
— mole (vomiting, hypertension, bleeding)
— hydramnios
— large baby (e.g. diabetes)

5. *Weight gain* should be 0.5 kg/week for the last 20 weeks.

The normal range is 0.2–0.9 kg/week.

Excessive weight gain suggests fluid retention.

Weight loss or weight gain of less than 0.5 kg/week for three consecutive weeks (assuming accurate weighing!) in the last trimester suggests placental insufficiency (in the absence of vomiting or deliberate dieting).

6. *The ultrasound scan* can identify the gestation sac (and therefore twins) at 6 weeks and the fetal heart at 7 weeks.

Estimations of gestation are more accurate early in pregnancy and are made by measuring:

— gestation sac — under 8 weeks
— crown-rump length — 8–11 weeks (accurate to 3 days at 9 weeks)
— biparietal diameter (BPD) — 13–20 weeks.

N.B. 12 weeks is a difficult time to estimate gestation by scan, falling between two measurements.

The BPD increases by about 3 mm/week at 20 weeks at 1 mm/week at term, up to about 95 mm. After 20 weeks, assessment of gestation by BPD becomes progressively inaccurate.

Fetal abdominal girth can be estimated and is useful in suspected placental insufficiency. A small increase relative to head circumference ('brain sparing') suggests loss of hepatic glycogen stores due to placental insufficiency.

The real-time ultrasound can detect most major anatomical abnormalities including neural tube defects, congenital heart lesions, diaphragmatic hernia, renal agenesis, urethral obstruction and intestinal obstruction.

7. The head is engaged when the widest diameter has passed through the brim of the pelvis. Clinically the head is usually just engaged when the UPPERMOST part of the fetal head that is palpable, (the occipital part) is at the level of the symphysis pubis. 1 cm higher than this is described as 3/5 (almost engaged) and 1 cm lower as 2/5 (engaged).

If the fetal head will pass through the pelvic brim it will certainly pass through the outlet (of a normally-shaped pelvis) because the outlet can be expanded by movement of the sacro-iliac joints and symphysis pubis.

Primips have an untried pelvis and in 30% of primips the head is still not engaged at 36 weeks but most will have a normal delivery. It can be due to a full rectum. Minor disproportion can be overcome by good contractions and moulding of the fetal head and the birth canal. In African women the head often appears high until late in labour.

Management of a high head after 36 weeks involves:

— scan (? placenta praevia, ? hydrocephalus)
— VE (? large cyst or fibroid)

The woman is allowed a trial of labour with full intrapartum monitoring. If labour fails to progress, section is performed.

True disproportion used to be common (due to rickets) but is now uncommon and usually due to:

— kyphoscoliosis; displaced pelvic fractures
— small stature — under 5 feet tall (152 cm)
— large baby (diabetes)

8. *Gestation* of pregnancy can be estimated from:

— LMP ('plus 7 minus 3' to estimate EDD, e.g. if LMP is 7.6.83 EDD is 14.3.84 An obstetric calender is better.).
— clinical examination (two examinations by an experienced doctor in the first 16 weeks can provide an accurate assessment)
— early scan (most accurate at 9 weeks)
— in later pregnancy estimation becomes more difficult
— L: S ratio (best method; above 2 means lungs are mature and producing surfactant and RDS is unlikely)
— rate of increase of BPD — (provides a clue to gestation, 1 mm per week suggesting near term)
— fetal knee X-ray (the lower femoral epiphysis is visible at 36 weeks, the upper tibial at 38 weeks)

Antenatal check-list   *First consultation (GP)*

— diagnosis of pregnancy
— dating conception
— appointment for booking examination (30 minutes)

The modern pregnancy testing kits detect the beta sub-unit of HCG and are very sensitive, some becoming positive before the first missed period (sometimes helpful in the diagnosis of ectopic pregnancy).

Booking (GP)

— Full history and examination
— MSU
— Blood tests

    — FBC
    — ABO and Rhesus
    — Rubella antibodies
    — WR and VDRL
    — Hepatitis B status
    — Sickling test (immigrants)

— Chest x-ray (immigrants)
— Discuss place of confinement
— Pattern of care (community, shared, specialist)
— Genetic counselling (if not given preconception)
— Parent craft classes
— Start shared-case card

16 weeks (GP)

— Routine observations weight, BP, MSU
— Fundal height (should be 6 cm above symphysis)
— Ultrasound scan (ideally for all):

    — confirm pregnancy (missed abortion, mole)
    — confirm dates by BPD estimation
    — multiple pregnancy identified
    — placenta praevia identified
    — gross abnormalities identified

— MSAFP (with consent)
— Indications for amniocentesis?
— Iron and vitamin supplements started

20 and 24 weeks (midwife)

— Routine observations (Fundus, WT, BP, MSU).

28 weeks (GP)

— Routine observations including oedema
— Fetal heart
— Check Hb
— Rhesus antibodies (if Rh negative)
— Uric acid (if previous PET. High means it will recur)
— Ultrasound scan

    — if any second trimester bleeding (? praevia)
    — if small for dates (? gestational age)
    — if large for dates (? multiple)

— Booking arrangements (? need changing)

30 and 32 weeks (midwife)

— routine observations

34 weeks (GP)

— routine observations
— malpresentation in nullip (refer)
— pre-eclampsia signs start at 34 weeks usually
— suspected growth retardation (refer for scan, oestriols etc)

    — poor weight gain
    — fundal height not increasing
    — diminished fetal movements

— Bloods

    — Check Hb
    — ABO and Rhesus (group and antibodies)
    — Hepatitis B status
    — uric acid (if history of PET)

36 weeks (GP)

— routine observations
— pelvic assessment in the nullip

    — avoid VE if any suspicion of praevia
    — head usually engaged in primip by 36 weeks
    — high head (? disproportion — refer)
    — pelvimetry if primip with breech

— consider a kick chart to monitor fetal well-being
— consider vaginal swabs for carriers if history of:

    — recurrent genital herpes (swab positive — ? section)
    — β-haemolytic streptococci (neonatal speticaemia)

37, 38 and 39 weeks (midwife)

— routine observations

40 weeks (GP)

— routine observations
— consider place for confinement

    — reducing movements — ? specialist unit
    — head not engaging — ? specialist unit

41 weeks (GP)

— routine observations
— reassess dates

    — PNM rises from 41 weeks
    — correlate information (fundal height, scans, movements)

— assess the cervix (by Bishop score):

Bishop score	0	1	2	3	Patient's score
Dilation of cervix (cms)	1	1–2	3–4	4	
Length of cervix (cms)	3	2–3	1–2	1	
Consistency of cervix	Firm	average	soft	—	
Position of cervix	posterior	central	anterior	—	
Level of presenting part	−3	−2	−1.0	+1, +2	

Total _____

A high score (above 10) suggests labour is imminent.
A low score (under 5) indicates induction may be difficult

    — plan for possible induction in specialist unit.

42 weeks (GP)

— plan for induction
— only allowed to continue if:

— dates uncertain
— low Bishop score
— normal CTG trace and movements

The concept of preventative antenatal care, suggested by Ballantyne at the turn of the century, became formalized over 50 years ago. Since then, the recommended schedule for visits has changed very little, (monthly to 28 weeks, fortnightly to 36, weekly to term). The aim is to detect serious complications of pregnancy and identify high-risk cases at booking. Recent studies (Chng, Hall and MacGillivray 1980) showed routine antenatal care had poor prognostic values with respect to the outcome of pregnancy. A revised system of antenatal care (Hall 1985) was no more effective. Devolving more care to the community was popular but did not reduce specialist workload. These studies emphasize that one of the main functions of antenatal care remains the providing of information, advice and reassurance which continue to be important although the benefits are hard to measure.

General advice

1. Most clinics run *antenatal classes* on infant feeding, clothing, parentcraft, bonding and education about pregnancy and labour. Knowing how to recognize labour and understanding what to expect decreases the fear and pain of labour.

Many women now also want to know about epidurals, pethidine, intrapartum monitoring and policies about episiotomy. Many couples also learn techniques of psycho-prophylaxis through such organizations as the National Childbirth Trust and their opinions about how they want to have their own baby must be respected (see Alternative Methods of Child-birth).

Antenatal exercises are directed towards present health and posture rather than preparation for child-birth.

Financial benefits; maternity allowances, free prescriptions, free dental treatment (see Documentation).

2. *Diet* Protein (100 g), calcium and iron intake should be increased — milk, cheese, eggs, meat and fresh vegetables. Carbohydrate need not be increased and 2400 calories per day is adequate. Constipation is a common problem and a high fluid intake and roughage are important.

3. High *alcohol* intake and heavy *smoking* both cause growth retardation and increased PNM

4. Most women stop *work* at 32 weeks. Normal daily activities should be continued although an afternoon rest is advisable in later pregnancy. Insommnia is a common problem in later pregnancy and mild hypnotics are safe, e.g. temazepam 10 mg.

5. *Sex* is not harmful at any time in pregnancy. However it is usual to forbid intercourse in:

— habitual abortion

— threatened abortion
— antepartum haemorrhage

6. *Drugs in Pregnancy*. It is well to remember the thalidomide disaster when discussing drugs in pregnancy. In 1960–61 in West Germany an outbreak of phocomelia occurred, eventually traced to the sedative thalidomide marketed there in 1956 as Contergan and in Britain in 1958 as Distaval. Taken between 5–8 weeks gestation it was teratogenic in about 20% of pregnancies. 5,000 deformed children survived in West Germany and 400 in Britain. The disaster resulted in the setting up of the Committee on Safety of Medicines.

Drug use in pregnancy has decreased considerably in the past twenty years. About 35% of women now take drugs in pregnancy, most commonly mild analgesics (17%), antibiotics (10%), and antacids (7%). Drugs such as anticonvulsants and bronchodilators, for which careful monitoring of dose is necessary, are prescribed in about 1% of pregnancies (increased liver metabolism of pregnancy means higher doses of these drugs are usually needed).

Drugs can harm the fetus at any stage of pregnancy. Drugs cross the placenta (a lipid barrier) by passive diffusion and although lipid soluble drugs pass across more rapidly, all drugs, given time, will achieve roughly equal concentration on each side of the placenta. The only notable exception is heparin (a large highly polar molecule).

In the first trimester there is the risk of teratogenesis and congenital malformation. The greatest risk if between 3–11 weeks. The drugs particularly linked with teratogenesis are cytotoxics (high risk), etretinate, lithium, podophyllin, phenytoin, valproate (neural tube defects), warfarin (limb defects, optic atrophy, deafness), trimetheprim (folate antagonist), quinine in high doses, progestagens to prevent abortion, alcohol and live vaccines. However no drug is safe beyond doubt in early pregnancy.

In the second and third trimesters some drugs have toxic effects on the fetus:

— sex hormones (virilization of female fetus)
— Thiazides (neonatal thrombocytomenia)
— Amiodarone (neonatal goitre)
— Iodides (neonatal goitre)
— Lithium (neonatal goitre)
— Warfarin (neonatal haemorrhage)
— Aspirin (closure of ductus)
— Indomethacin (closure of ductus)
— Streptomycin (deafness)
— Chloramphenicol (vascular collapse)
— Tetracycline (discoloured teeth)
— Sulphonamides (Kernicterus)
— Dapsone (neonatal haemolysis)

Some drugs, e.g. ketoconazole, are toxic in animal studies and best avoided. Stimulant laxatives may precipitate premature labour in sensitive individuals.

Drugs given shortly before labour can effect labour or affect the neonate after delivery:

— Verapamil, nifedipine (may inhibit labour)
— Salbutamol in high doses (delayed labour)
— Benzodiazepines (depress respiration; withdrawal symptoms)
— Tricyclic antidepressants (neonatal irritability, fits)
— Aminophylline (neonatal apnoea)

Drugs that can be safely prescribed in pregnancy:

— Antacids (magnesium with aluminium salts to avoid bowel disturbance. Low sodium content to avoid fluid retention.)
— Iron and folic acid (e.g. Pregaday — ferrous fumarate 304 mg equivalent to 100 mg elemental iron and 350 g folic acid)
— Water soluble vitamins (e.g. Pregnavite forte)
— Penicillins, Cephalosporins, Erythromycin
— Paracetamol
— Short-acting benzodiazepines (temazepam, oxazepam)

Minor symptoms
— Nausea
— Heartburn
— Breathlessness
— Headaches
— Oedema
— Constipation
— Vaginal discharge
— Varicose veins
— Haemorrhoids
— Cramps
— Itching
— Carpal tunnel syndrome
— Backache

1. *Nausea* occurs in most pregnancies in the early weeks, usually, but not always, in the mornings. It is often reduced by a small meal. It is temporary and resolves around 14–16 weeks. Drugs should be avoided unless it is seriously interfering with lifestyle. Antihistamines are generally recommended for treating severe nausea and vomiting. Cyclizine is widey used and safe. Debendox (a combination of dicyclomine, doxylamine and pyridoxine) was withdrawn by the manufacturers in 1983 because of unsubstantiated claims about teratogenicity. For the management for severe nausea or vomiting see the section on Hyperemesis Gravidarum.

2. *Heartburn* is common in pregnancy probably due to relaxation of the oesophageal and pyloric sphincters with reflux of bile and acid. Increased progesterone and reduced motilin levels are thought to be responsible. Pressure from the uterine

fundus in late pregnancy may aggravate the problem. Simple measures include:

— raising the bed-head
— avoid large meals
— avoid stooping or straining
— loose-fitting clothes

Antacids can safely be used, e.g. aluminium hydroxide. Cimetidine and metoclopramide have not been widely used in pregnancy and should be avoided.

3. *Breathlessness* occurs in 50% and can occur early in gestation. It is probably due to a combination of the physiological hyperventilation of pregnancy (a progesterone effect, lowering material CO_2 hence easier transfer of fetal CO_2) together with the 30% increase in cardiac output by 12 weeks so maximal output is reached at relatively low levels of activity. It is important to examine and exclude lung and heart disease and to consider the possibility of diffuse pulmonary emboli before explaining and reassuring.

4. *Headaches*. Tension headaches can be safely treated with paracetamol 1 g every 4–6 hours. Avoid aspirin (haemostatic abnormalities, delayed labour) and diazepam (neonatal withdrawal symptoms). Migraine sufferers often notice a fall in frequency of attacks. If migraine occurs treat with paracetamol and an antiemetic such as prochlorperazine. Consider precipitating factors. Propranolol 40 mg BD is effective prophylaxis for 60%. Ergotamine tartrate is usually withheld but it is not in fact oxytocic and if it is the only effective remedy for an individual it can be prescribed sparingly.

5. *Oedema* of the legs is common due to a combination of fluid retention (6–8 litres of water and 500–800 mEq of sodium) and venous obstruction by the gravid uterus. It is worse in the obese or with varicose veins. Elevation of the legs (above the level of the right atrium) will reduce swelling. Exclude PET (especially if swelling is rapid or generalized) and advise support stockings. Diuretics should not be given.

6. *Constipation* affects at least 30% and may be aggravated by haemorrhoids. Colonic transit time is increased, probably an effect of progesterone. Iron often increases constipation. Encourage a high fluid, high fibre diet. Prescribe faecal softeners for severe constipation, but avoid stimulant laxatives, (uterine contractions in sensitive individuals) mineral oils (malabsorption of fat soluble vitamins?) and small bowel purgatives (electrolyte imbalance).

7. *Vaginal discharge*. Increased leucorrhoea is physiological in pregnancy and the woman may need explanation and re-assurance. Smell, itching or soreness are pathological and indicate HVS and endocervical swabs. The common pathogens are *Candida*, *Trichomonas*, but remember gonorrhoea. Clotri-

mazole, econazole and metronidazole all seem to be safe in pregnancy.

8. *Varicose Veins* (legs and vulva) tend to worsen in pregnancy but treatment should be conservative because they regress on delivery.

9. *Haemorrhoids* are common in pregnancy. Avoid constipation and if necessary soften the stools (e.g. Diocytl sodium 100 mg b.d.). Treat conservatively if possible with astringent suppositories (e.g. Anusol) and analgesic ointment (e.g. Nupercaine). Thrombosed perianal haematomas can be incised under local anaesthetic. Injection or ligation of haemorrhoids in pregnancy is usually unsuccessful because of the large numbers of dilated vessels. Ligation may be considered in the puerperium.

10. *Cramps* are a common complaint. No disturbances of sodium or calcium metabolism has been demonstrated. Calcium and vitamin D supplements are no more effective than placebo. Quinine has a low teratogenic risk but is often ineffective in pregnancy. Reassurance, explanation and instruction on passive stretching and massage are important.

11. *Itching*. Troublesome itching occurs in about 1% of pregnancies. Consider liver function tests to look for cholestasis of pregnancy. Itching interferes with sleep and treatment should aim at a good night's sleep. Aqueous cream as a soap substitute can help. Antihistamines have a sedative effect and are best given at night e.g. chlorpheniramine (Piriton) 8 mg nocte.

12. *Carpal tunnel syndrome* occurs in about 5% of pregnancies, tingling and pain that can radiate up the forearm characteristically waking the woman at night. Sensory loss or wasting indicate long term compression and other causes should be sought. A mild diuretic often helps — e.g. Moduretic (5 mg amiloride plus 50 mg hydrochlorothiazide). Night splints or local steroid injection may be preferred. Surgical decompression is usually unnecessary during pregnancy, because the symptoms often stop after delivery.

13. *Backache* is common due to softening of connective tissues and exaggerated lumbar lordosis and strain. Advise the woman to avoid high heels and excessive backward-leaning and to sleep on a firm mattress. Light massage by the physiotherapist can be helpful. Mild analgesics are harmless e.g. paracetamol. Non-steroidal anti-inflammatory drugs should be avoided (closure of ductus and delayed labour). Aspirin should be avoided in pregnancy (crosses the placenta and causes reduced platelet function).

Amniocentesis Performed at 16 weeks (when an adequate sample is obtainable) to detect fetal abnormality but only if the woman would accept a termination. Ultrasound is necessary to localize the placenta, to confirm gestation (needed to interpret the results) and to exclude obvious abnormality. Anti-D (50 μg) is given if the woman is Rhesus negative. The abortion rate is 1%. *The indications are*:

1. Maternal age is over 40
2. Previous baby with Down's syndrome
3. Previous baby with neural tube defect (spina bifida, anencephaly, hydrocephaly)
4. EH (first degree relative with these abnormalities)
5. Mother is carrier of X-linked disorder, (haemophilia; Duchenne muscular dystrophy) — 50% of male infants will be affected
6. Previous baby with inborn error of metabolism (e.g. Tay-Sachs disease) — recessive, therefore 25% chance of recurrence

It may be performed on request for *lower risk situations*, e.g. mother over 35 or a history of recurrent abortions or unexplained stillbirths.

Fluid analysis for AFP or sex chromatin determination takes 24 hours. Cell culture for karyotype or biochemistry takes 3 weeks.

The risks of Down's syndrome are:

Age 35+	0.5%
Age 40+	1%
Age 45+	2%

(Amniocentesis is also performed from 26 weeks in cases of rhesus immunization to measure bilirubin concentration and around 36 weeks to assess fetal maturity by L:S ratio, prior to induction).

Prenatal diagnosis Antenatal diagnosis of congenital or inherited disease is based on imaging techniques. (see section on the ultrasound scan), or the laboratory analysis of fetal material.

Techniques for obtaining antenatal material include:

— amniocentesis
— chorionic villus biopsy
— fetoscopy
— cordocentesis

Techniques for analysis fetal material include:

— chromosome analysing (Karyotyping)
— enzyme assay
— gene probe technology to analyse DNA

Screening of maternal serum AFP increases the detection rate of some congenital abnormalities.

Chorionic Villus Biopsy (CVB)

The first report of CVB was in 1973 using a small hysteroscope and biopsy forceps. The development of DNA analysis for fetal diagnosis (particular for the haemoglobinopathies) provided the impetus to develop a safe simple method of obtaining chorionic villus material early in pregnancy. Aspiration techniques under ultrasound control were introduced in 1983.

Chorionic villus biopsy (CVB) is carried out at 9–11 weeks gestation (after the period of rapid embryonic development and organogenesis is over).

The aim is to obtain villi without puncturing the amniotic sac. The advantages of CVB over amniocentesis are:

a) Direct analysis of tissue is possible without the need for cell culture (and hence less delay in diagnosis) and only a few villi are needed to provide enough material for analysis.
b) If termination is required it can be carried out in the first trimester.

Technique: Villi are aspirated from the placental edge under real-time ultrasound scan control via a soft cannula that is passed either transcervically or transabdominally. The success rate is improved by facilities for microscopy in theatre, so the biopsy can be repeated if the frond-like villi are not seen in the sample. The abortion rate is around 3% for the transcervical route, most abortions occurring 3–4 weeks later, probably due to chlamydial infection picked up from the cervix, therefore the transabdominal route may prove safer.

Rhesus negative women should be given an injection of 100 μg of anti-1gD.

Fetoscopy

Fetoscopy is feasible after 18 weeks gestation and causes fetal loss in around 3%. The indications for fetal blood sampling are dwindling with the advent of chorionic villus biopsy, and newer techniques for blood sampling under ultrasound control will probably supersede fetoscopy where fetal blood sampling is still required. Fetal blood (taken from placental vessels) can be used to diagnose:

— sickle cell disease
— thalassaemia (and other haemoglobinopathies)
— haemophilia
— immune deficiency syndromes

Assays of factor 8 and 9 are possible, and assay for beta-globin chains (but only after 18 weeks).

Fetoscopy can also be used for:

— skin biopsy (epidermolysis bullosa lethalis)
— liver biopsy (urea cycle enzyme deficiencies)
— rapid Karyotyping.

Cordocentesis

Fetal blood samples can be obtained from the umbilical cord either fetoscopically or by means of an ultrasound guided needle.

The traditional indications for sampling are the pre-natal diagnosis of genetic disorders and the management of rhesus disease. More recently it has been used for Karyotyping of fetuses during the third trimester with correctable malformations and to evaluate abnormal CTG traces in labour. It has also been used to diagnose fetal hypoxia and acidosis in IUGR.

Chromosomal abnormalities

Most chromosomal abnormalities result in first trimester abortions, or multiple congenital abnormalities with death soon after birth. Some chromosomal abnormalities compatible with survival are:

— Trisomy 21 (Down's syndrome)
— Trisomy 18
— Trisomy 13
— Monosomy XO (Turner's syndrome)
— Triple X XXX (Mental retardation)
— Fragile X syndrome (Mental retardation)

97% of trisomies are due to non-dysjunction, with only a 1.5% recurrence risk following an abnormal child. 3% of trisomies are due to a balanced translocation in the mother, with 25% chance of recurrence.

These monosomies and trisomies can be diagnosed directly on chorionic villus preparations. More subtle anomalies (inversions, small deletions) require detailed banding best obtained from cultured cells.

Enzyme assays

There are about 200 inherited diseases due to a single enzyme defects. Many of these inborn errors of metabolism can be diagnosed by incubation of fetal tissue with a specific substrate.

Enzyme assay is indicated for known carriers or if there has been a previously affected child. Some of the more common enzyme deficiencies include

— Tay-Sachs disease (β-D-hexosaminidase)
— Niemann Pick disease (Sphingomyelinase)
— Hurler's syndrome (β-D-glucuronidase)
— Gaucher's disease (β-D-glucosidase)
— Krabbe's disease (β-D-galactosidase)

There is rapid progress in this field and the medical genetics laboratory should be consulted before counselling a couple.

Gene Probe Technology

DNA technology has become so refined that the only 5 μg of DNA are required for each analysis (10 ml amniotic fluid or a single chorionic villus). DNA technology has only been clinically used to diagnose haemoglobinopathy in an at-risk fetus. However gene markers are now recognized for many genetic diseases which will be detectable prenatally by DNA analysis on chorionic villi.

The gene probe is a technique for recognizing fragments of DNA. The principle is that a fragment of DNA of known sequence is radio-labelled (the diagnostic probe) and then mixed with unknown DNA and it will stick to identical strands of DNA (hybridization) which can then be isolated by the technique of *Southern blotting*.

Gene probes of known sequence are made by means of restriction enzymes (extracted from bacteria) which cut DNA at particular nucleotide sequences. Having obtained the DNA in which one is interested (e.g. from a virus or a human chromosome) it can be replicated by inserting it into an E coli plasmid (a circle of DNA within the bacteria). Unknown DNA fragments of different restriction lengths (and therefore molecular weights) are separated on agarose gel by electrophoresis. They can then be isolated by blotting them with nitrocellulose paper which is porous and sucks the DNA fragments from the gel (a technique described in 1975 by E. Southern). A radio-labelled DNA probe is then added. This hybridizes with any identical DNA which can then be detected by autoradiography. One advantage of this method is that viruses can still be identified when they cannot be isolated in pure culture (e.g. human wart virus in tissue from cancer of the cervix, rotaviruses in faeces and Coxsackie B in myocardial biopsies in myocarditis).

Disorders with genetic markers detectable by DNA marker probes include:

— Thalassaemia (α and β)
— Sickle cell disease and trait
— Haemophilia and Christmas disease
— Adult polycystic kidney
— Lethal osteogenesis imperfecta
— Huntington's chorea
— Myotonic dystrophy
— Cystic fibrosis
— Muscular dystrophy (Ducterre and Becker)
— Lesch-Wylan syndrome
— Phenylketonuria

Fetal tissue is obtained by CVB around 12 weeks.

It is only a matter of years before all the genes responsible for diseases where the biochemical cause is known are cloned. It will then be possible to make DNA probes and diagnose the disorder by direct analysis of the DNA structure of fetal cells.

Fetal Therapy   A few medical and surgical abnormalities may be correctable before birth. Metabolic derangements may be treatable by manipulation of maternal diet or intra-amniotic installatios of nutrients. Simple structural defects may be correctable in utero. NTDs, craniostenoses, diaphragmatic hernia, hydrorephrosis and hydrocephalus are potential candidates. The treatment of these conditions is currently under investigation in animal models. Cardiac or renal transplantation in utero may become possible before the development of immune competence thereby abolishing the risk of rejection. Orofacial wounds in monkey fetuses heal within 24 hours with minimal evidence of tissue disruption, raising the possibility of intra-uterine repair of cleft lip and palate. (See also the section on the Ultrasound Scan.)

Maternal Serum AFP (MSAFP)

The incidence of NTDs ranges from 2–6 per 1000 in different parts of the country. Screening for maternal serum alpha-fetoprotein (MSAFP) is currently performed at 16–18 weeks for about 50% of pregnancies in Britain. AFP was first reported in fetal serum in 1956 and was first used for the prenatal diagnosis of spina bifida in 1972 when Brock and Sutcliffe demonstrated increased levels in amniotic fluid. In 1974 Wold reported that NTDs also caused raised AFP levels in maternal serum. 95% of NTD births are completely unsuspected, therefore a screening technique is valuable.

Accurate dating is important to interpret results correctly. MSAFP rises steadily throughout the second trimester. Assay of MSAFP is expressed in ng/ml but the normal range varies with gestational age and from lab to lab, therefore MSAFP levels are expressed in terms of multiples of the median (MoM), the cut off being between 2–3, above which action is required (i.e. ultrasound scan and possibly amniocentesis).

Screening will identify 85–90% of anencephaly and 60–80% open spina bifida, depending on the cut-off selected for action. In low incidence areas it may be necessary to use a higher cut-off to avoid subjecting too many patients to unnecessary amnio-centesis. 20% of spina bifida lesions are closed — i.e. skin-covered, and do not exude AFP.

Open ventral wall defects (gastroschisis and exomphalos) occur in 1 in 3000 pregnancies, and MSAFP is consistently elevated. 80–90% will be detected by screening.

Low levels of MSAFP occur in insulin-dependent diabetics, who have an increased risk of NTD pregnancies, therefore the cut-off needs to be adjusted in diabetics.

Women carrying Down's syndrome pregnancies have lower than average AFPs (although the difference between affected and unaffected populations in much less than for NTDs). A low MSAFP may be an indication for amniocentesis to exclude Down's syndrome.

Raised MSAFP occurs when AFP in fetal serum leaks into the maternal circulation. MSAFP is raised in:

— Open NTDs
— Multiple pregnancy
— Feto-maternal haemorrhage
— Fetal distress or death
— Open Ventral Wall defects.

A scan is indicated to check gestational age and fetal viability and identify twins or NTD. If BPD is larger than expected by the date of the LMP the MSAFP level is re-interpreted and may then fall within the normal level. If no explanation is found amniocentesis is indicated, to measure AFP in amniotic fluid.

Screening specificity is improved by allowing for maternal weight. Small women tend to have higher levels of MSAFP because fetal AFP is diluted by a smaller maternal circulating volume.

The ultrasound scan

The transducer or probe emits a narrow focussed beam of high frequency (2 to 5 MH^z) sound waves and records the return echoes. These are presented in a 'grey scale' format which produces an identifiable image. Fluid filled spaces (vessels, ducts, bladder, cysts) are echo-free because there are no interfaces to reflect the beam. The beam will not pass through gas therefore a window is sought through the bowel loops by using the full bladder or liver.

Ultrasound is high-pitched sound that is propagated through air and tissue by waves of compression and rarefaction The dissipation of this energy may result in heat, but heating or movement of body cells does not occur with diagnostic ultrasound, which is pulsed, so ultrasound energy is only delivered for one hundredth of the time of the examination (the rest of the time is spent 'listening' for returning echoes). It has no effect on DNA at diagnostic levels and has not been shown to be hazardous, but the early misuse of obstetric radiography reminds us not to be complacent.

Its main uses in obstetrics are for:

— diagnosis of pregnancy (? viable ? ectopic ? mole)
— establishing gestational age
— detection of multiple pregnancy
— placental localization
— monitoring fetal growth in diabetes
— assessing a small or large for dates fetus
— adjunct to other diagnostic procedures
— diagnosing congenital anomalies
— assessing presentation and lie

Notes

1. The ultrasound scan is useful in *early pregnancy* if there is pain and bleeding (? ectopic) or if there is severe vomiting (? twins ? mole), or if pregnancy was induced by fertility drugs (? multiple).

2. *Establishing gestational age.* Ultrasound is superior to pelvic examination in determining gestational age and is of proven value in those patients with unreliable menstrual histories (25%). The EDD estimated by the BPD measurement on ultrasound is more accurate (before 24 weeks) than using the date of the LMP. The BPD estimate is accurate to within one week, so if it disagrees with the menstrual history the ultrasound estimation should be used.

3. *Detection of multiple pregnancy.* Routine scanning has

reduced the mean time of diagnosis of twins from 36 to 20 weeks with a tenfold reduction in perinatal mortality due to failure to expect the second twin (sometimes until after the syntometrine has been given).

4. *Placental localization* can be performed from 16 weeks. 95% have a fundal placenta with no risk of a placenta praevia. The other 5% are scanned again at 32 weeks to identify the 0.5% that remain praevia.

5. *Diagnosis of growth retardation.* Symmetrical growth retardation (i.e. both BPD and abdominal circumference reduced) is usually due to a normal baby at the lower end of the normal range. Viral infections (TORCH infections — Toxoplasma, Rubella, Cytomegalovirus, Herpes) and congenital anomalies should be excluded and monitoring for continued fetal growth continued.

Assymetrical IUGR (a rise in Head/Abdominal circumference) is due to placental insufficiency and full monitoring with CTG_1 oestriols and kick chart is indicated to time delivery and avoid stillbirth or fetal distress in labour. Delivery is indicated if growth of the head stops.

6. *Diagnosing congenital abnormality.* A large number of abnormalities (CNS, heart, renal tract, abdominal wall, bowel and skeleton) can now be diagnosed antenatally. Indications for referral for high resolution ultrasound include:

— suspicious findings on routine scan
— small fetus
— previous child with anomaly
— family history of anomaly
— raised MSAFP
— prior to amniocentesis
— poly- or oligohydramnios
— exposure to teratogen
— maternal diabetes
— preterm labour (especially if breech)

The antenatal diagnosis of fetal abnormalities presents problems. Intrauterine surgery is limited to drainage procedures for obstructive uropathy (due to urethral valves) and hydrocephalus. Babies with cardiac abnormalities, diaphragmatic hernia, gastroschisis and exomphalos may benefit from transfer in utero to an obstetric unit with a neonatal surgical unit. The place of preterm delivery in all these anomalies is still being assessed. 2% of babies are born with a congenital abnormality. The antenatal diagnosis of an abnormality produces tremendous anxiety in the parents and may result in rejection of the baby at birth. For some major defects the benefits of knowing include prompt treatment on delivery. In many cases the extent of the lesion is uncertain and if termination is declined or is impossible the couple face increasing anxiety until delivery. Although errors are rare the consequences are considerable and, if termination is advised in error, disastrous. The management of this situation involves good communication between the whole team of professionals involved.

7. Seeing the baby on a scan is an emotional experience for most parents. Mother's who have seen a scan are more likely to give up smoking and alcohol and attend antenatal clinics regularly.

Antenatal monitoring

Antenatal monitoring of the fetus involves:

— a fetal movement chart
— CTG (3 × per week)
— serial oestriols (3 × per week)
— serial HPL levels
— serial scans (fortnightly)

Monitoring is indicated from 28 weeks (i.e. from the time the fetus is normally viable) in conditions associated with intra-uterine death:

— small-for-dates
— conditions associated with placental insufficiency (pre-eclampsia, hypertension, chronic renal failure, APH post-maturity and twins).
— diabetes
— rhesus antibodies
— previous perinatal death

Notes

1. *Fetal movements* probably cease about 48 hours before intra-uterine death occurs. Observations by the patient on the activity of her fetus are a simple and reliable measure of fetal wellbeing. In one method (the kick chart) the woman notes the time each day by when she has counted 10 fetal movements (not just 'kicks') starting at 9 am. However some women don't notice fetal movements and others sometimes become over-anxious using this method.

If the woman has felt no movements for 12 hours, she attends for a CTG.

2. *The cardiotocograph (CTG)* is a continuous recording of the fetal heart rate and rhythm (using an external amplifier) and of maternal contractions (using a tocometer).

It is performed 2–3 × per week (or sometimes daily as an inpatient) for 10–20 minutes and gives an indication of fetal wellbeing. A normal trace is taken to imply fetal wellbeing for the next 48 hours.

A flat trace (poor beat-to-beat variation) with no accelerations in heart rate on fetal movement (non-reactive trace) indicates chronic hypoxia. If other tests are also poor (few movements, falling oestrogens, poor growth rate) induction is considered.

A very poor trace (e.g. unprovoked dips) can be an indication for emergency section.

Long distance telemetry is possible using a portable ultra-sound fetal heart rate detector (e.g. Sonicaid). The mouthpiece of a telephone is held to the loudspeaker and the recording undergoes real-time processing by a computer in the obstetric department. This can save some women who need daily moni-toring from prolonged admission.

3. *Oestriol* is produced by the feto-placental unit (see physiology of pregnancy) and serial measurements on 24-hour urine show a steady rise throughout pregnancy although there is a wide normal variation. Plasma levels can now be measured by radioimmunoassay.

Very low levels occur in intra-uterine death, anencephaly, high-dose steroid therapy, antibiotic therapy and the rare placental sulphatase deficiency (about 1 in 5000–10 000. Diagnosed by sulphated oestrogen precursors in the urine — detected by chromatography. Associated with prolonged labour due to poor cervical softening and with icthyosis in male infants due to the same enzyme defect). Low levels also occur in diabetes and rhesus isoimmunization when monitoring oestriols is of little value. High levels occur with twins.

One low reading is meaningless but if serial measurements plotted on a graph fall below the lower limit of normal, it may indicate placental failure. Alternatively with a borderline scan the oestriols may indicate that it is safe to allow the pregnancy to continue.

4. *Human placental lactogen (HPL)* resembles growth hormone. It is secreted by the trophoblast from 5 weeks and rises gradually to term correlating closely with placental weight.

It causes breast growth and, like growth hormone, is dia-betogenic (lipolysis and peripheral resistance to insulin).

Serial plasma levels (radioimmunoassay) are used as a test of placental function.

5. *Fortnightly ultrasound scans* monitor fetal growth by measuring BPD and abdominal girth. Placental insufficiency affects the abdominal girth, (decreased liver glycogen) before it affects the growth of the head (brain sparing) as measured by serial BPD estimation. The BPD increases by about 3 mm per week at 20 weeks and at 1 mm per week at term. At least a fortnight is needed between scans to monitor growth rate. One estimation is of little help because fetal size *obviously* varies.

N.B. These tests are used together as a guide to the condition of the fetus. It is the overall pattern that dictates action (induction or section) and not individual results.

Note that changes in fetal wellbeing are detected over different time-scales by different methods:

— CTG — hours
— kick chart — hours
— oestriols — days
— scans — weeks

Placental insufficiency

Growth retardation is first detectable clinically at 28 weeks (by fundal height and fetal size). Placental insufficiency never occurs before 28 weeks because the placental reserve is too great (it weights 4 × as much as the fetus at 10 weeks but only a third at 28 weeks).

The PNM is increased due to intra-uterine hypoxia and intrapartum anoxia ad it is now the major cause of perinatal death apart from congenital abnormalities.

Features suggesting placental insufficiency are:

1. Poor weight gain. Less than 0.5 kg/week for 3 weeks — (breasts, fat, fetus, placenta are all affected by placental hormones, and therefore weight reflects placental function).

2. Small-for-dates. The fundal height above the symphysis should be only 3 cm less than the gestation in weeks. In addition there may be oligohydramnios. Admit to confirm gestation, exclude fetal abnormality and monitor the fetus (see fetal monitoring).

3. Decreasing fetal movements

Since only 50% of cases are detectable clinically, patients with a high risk of IUGR should also be monitored. *Factors associated with growth retardation are*:

— age over 35
— parity (first or fifth baby)
— social class 5
— height less than 5 feet (152 cm)
— heavy smoking or drinking
— previous IUGR
— severe anaemia
— twins
— conditions associated with placental insufficiency:

  — PET
  — hypertension
  — chronic renal failure
  — APH

Management involves the following:

— confirm the dates (i.e. exclude the wrong dates)
— admit to monitor the fetus
— deliver in a unit with attached SCBU
— postpone delivery as long as the fetal condition is satisfactory, then decide between induction or section
— monitor in labour
— short controlled second stage is indicated for vaginal delivery. Avoid pethidine.
— suck out any meconium from the pharynx at birth and monitor blood sugars for 72 hours by Dextrostix.

The baby's weight will be below the 10th centile for its

gestational age, and such a light-for-dates (dysmature) infant has a 4 × increase in neonatal death rate from:

— meconium aspiration
— hypoglycaemia
— hypothermia

Pre-eclampsia (PET)

A syndrome of

— oedema
— hypertension (above 140/90)
— proteinuria (above 0.3 g/l per 24 hours)

Pre-eclampsia rarely occurs before 30 weeks and is seen in 5–10% of pregnancies. The patient is usually a primip and it is more likely to develop if she is over 35, obese or already hypertensive. It is unlikely to recur in her subsequent pregnancies (recurs in 15%). There is an increased PNM and maternal mortality. The dangers are:

— placental insufficiency (death or IUGR)
— placental abruption (rare)
— eclamptic fits
— acute renal failure
— cerebral haemorrhage
— DIC (very rare)

The cause is unknown, but it is seen more commonly in conditions associated with a large placenta (twins, mole, hydrops, diabetes) and can appear or worsen in the 48 hours after delivery.

Possibly a placental vasoactive substance causes vasoconstriction (hypertension and organ ischaemia) and increased vessel permeability (hypovolaemia and oedema). At post-mortem there are scattered cerebral and hepatic haemorrhages, swollen glomeruli and DIC.

Management

1. The key to good management is early detection. *Oedema* occurs in all pregnancies and therefore is the least important sign. It is generalized (pretibial, face, fingers) and causes excessive weight gain (1 kg/week). With marked oedema, increase the antenatal visits to monitor the BP. Diuretics do not alter the course of PET and should be avoided.

2. Admit for bedrest if *hypertension* develops (BP above 140/90 or a rise in diastolic of more than 20 mmHg from booking). Bedrest:

— lowers the BP
— improves placental blood flow
— can cause a diuresis

Exclude other causes of hypertension (MSU, U & E, possibly 24-hour VMA) and *monitor the pre-eclampsia*:

— 4-hourly BP
— 24-hour protein excretion
— creatinine clearance
— serial uric acid levels (may rise)
— serial platelet counts (may fall)

Fetal wellbeing is monitored (see antenatal monitoring).

Usually the BP settles down in a few days and the woman is allowed home and monitored regularly in the antenatal clinic (or by the district midwife). Fetal monitoring must continue.

3. Re-admission is indicated if:

— BP rises above 140/90
— proteinuria develops (a sign that PET is out of control)
— weight gain or oedema are excessive
— there is evidence of IUGR

Management involves:

— monitoring (weight, BP, proteinuria)
— monitoring the fetus
— group and save serum (emergency section)

Labour is usually induced at 38 weeks or earlier of the pre-eclampsia or fetal condition are worsening. The development of proteinuria is a serious sign and often signals a worsening of the condition.

Methyl-dopa is not started in late pregnancy as it probably worsens placental function. Pre-eclampsia resolves on delivery and the treatment for severe pre-eclampsia is induction. After delivery the condition usually resolves rapidly (although during the first 24 hours it occasionally worsens).

4. Signs of severe pre-eclampsia and impending fits (*eclampsia*) are:

— headaches
— blurred vision (retinal ischaemia)
— nausea and epigastric pain (hepatic haemorrhages)
— hyper reflexia (test the biceps)
— twitching
— rapid rise in BP

Management involves:

— avoid noise and bright lights (which may precipitate fits)
— i.v. chlormethiazole (anticonvulsant — keep well sedated)
— i.v. hydrallazine (aim for diastolic of 90)
— epidural (pain can precipitate fits, also epidural lowers the diastolic 10–20 mmHg)
— induce labour (with full intrapartum monitoring)
— catheterize (give i.v. manitol or frusemide if urine output falls below 30 ml/hour)
— keep sedated until at least 12 hours after delivery

Section is performed if progress is slow or fetal distress develops.

Under 34 weeks emergency section is usually performed because induction is difficult and fetal distress more likely.

Hypertension

1. The BP falls in pregnancy, especially in the middle trimester (the systolic by about 10 mmHg and the diastolic by about 20 mmHg) due to vasodilation and the low resistance of the placental circulation.

2. BP above 140/90 in the first 24 weeks of pregnancy implies the existence of hypertension before pregnancy and occurs in about 1%. About 30% of such women develop pre-eclampsia (a further rise in BP with oedema and proteinuria).

3. BP above 170/100 increases the fetal loss to 30% due to accelerated placental degeneration and an increased risk of placental abruption. The maternal risks are LVF or cerebral haemorrhage.

4. *Any cause* for the hypertension must be excluded:

— renal disease (MSU, U & E)
— renal artery stenosis (abdominal systolic bruit)
— co-arctation (decreased and delayed femoral pulses)
— phaeochromocytoma (24-hour urinary V.M.A.)
— Hydatidiform mole (ultrasound scan)

And the duration assessed:

— fundi (A-V nipping, haemorrhages, exudates, papilloedema)
— LVH (apex beat, CXR, ECG)

5. *Management* involves:

— bedrest and monitor the BP. Often this is enough to control the BP, particularly as it falls in the middle trimester. If not:
— Methyldopa (initially 250 mg BD) is known to be safe and effective in pregnancy and does not adversely effect the fetal growth. Aim for a diastolic of 90 mmHg (maternal hypotension can cause fetal death). It does not prevent pre-eclampsia from developing. Propranolol is also widely used. Good control of hypertension reduces PNM.
— Monitor the fetus. Induce at 38 weeks or earlier if the fetal condition is deteriorating (after L:S ratio). Section would be performed if delivery was necessary before 36 weeks.
— Lifelong follow-up is necessary.

Diabetes

Diabetes is associated with an increased PNM due to an increased incidence of:

— congenital abnormalities ($\times 4$)
— intra-uterine death (? cause)
— long labour (large baby)
— RDS

With good control there is no increase in the incidence of a big baby, hydramnios, pre-eclampsia or UTI. Clinically there are two distinct situations:

1. Gestational diabetes
2. Pregnancy in a known diabetic

Gestational diabetes

This is symptomless but increases the PNM to around 5% (50 per 1000). It is suspected if there are any potential diabetic features:

— glycosuria ×2 (10% will have an abnormal GTT)
— obesity
— FH of diabetes (in first degree relative)
— previous gestational diabetes
— previous big baby (10 lb or 4.5 kg)
— previous unexplained PNM
— RDS or hypoglycaemia in previous babies
— hydramnios

N.B. Glycosuria in early pregnancy is more likely to be due to diabetes than threshold changes. Test an early morning specimen to avoid postprandial glycosuria.

However 30% of patients with gestational diabetes do not have these features, therefore a glucose load test is now advocated at booking and at 32 weeks to screen for gestational diabetes. A 50 g glucose drink is taken (non-fasting) and a blood test taken 1 hour later. Levels above 7.5 mmol/l indicate the need for a full GTT.

The 75 g oral GTT is recommended. A diagnosis of impaired glucose tolerance is made if (venous) glucose levels are above:

5.5 mmol/l — fasting
12.5 mmol/l — 1 hour
9.5 mmol/l — 2 hours
7.5 mmol/l — 3 hours

N.B. The blood glucose levels in pregnancy should be normal — fasting glucose is a bit lower and the peak after glucose a bit higher.

Management of impaired glucose tolerance involves:

— Blood sugar series on a normal diet. Preprandial glucose estimations throughout one day. If the average exceeds 5.5 mmol/l, treatment is indicated.
— 150 g CHO diet with high fibre. Repeat blood sugar series. If still above 5.5 mmol/l, insulin is indicated.
— Human Ultratard (10 units daily) is started and blood glucose monitored. If glucose peaks occur a BD regime with Actrapid is added.
— Monitor the fetus
— Induce at 38 weeks (increased incidence of intrauterine death towards term).

Oral hypoglycaemic agents are avoided in pregnancy. They cross the placenta and may provoke fetal hyperinsulinaemia.

The blood glucose levels return to normal within 48 hours of delivery (as cortisol and HPL levels fall). The woman needing insulin has an increased risk of developing diabetes (about 20% at 5 years, rising with each pregnancy), therefore follow-up is important.

The known diabetic

Before the introduction of insulin in 1922 maternal mortality for diabetics was 30% and 90% of babies died in utero.

Poor control of diabetes still causes many complications for mother and baby, and PNM can rise to 30% (Ketoacidosis is rapidly lethal to the fetus), whereas with perfect control (normal HbA_{Ic} levels) the risks are probably no greater than for non-diabetics. With home glucose monitoring admission to hospital is no longer necessary providing control is perfect and the pregnancy is normal. It is obviously essential that care is shared between the obstetrician and diabetic specialist in a joint clinic.

1. *Preconception*. The diabetic woman should be advised to start her family early, partly because of her decreased life expectancy and because PNM becomes very high if she develops complications (nephropathy, retinopathy). Her pregnancy should be planned and HbA_{Ic} (glycosylated Hb) levels must be checked before stopping contraception (levels above 10% may significantly increase the chances of congenital abnormality).

Glycosylated Hb falls in *normal* pregnancy from 9% to 3% due to increased FBC production. The aim should be to see the same fall in the well-controlled diabetic.

2. *Antenatal care*. She should book early for antenatal care in a unit with an attached SCBU. An accurate assessment of gestation (early scan) is important for timing delivery and to implement good control of the diabetes. The motivation in these women is high and excellent diabetic control can be achieved with home monitoring using blood testing strips (e.g. Dextrostix, BM Test, Visidex) together with a reflectance meter (e.g. Glucocheck, Glucometer, Hypocount). The aim is to keep preprandial plasma glucose below 6 mmol/l. In about a third of women the morning result is high (morning surge of cortisol and growth hormone) and yet increasing the teatime dose tends to cause nocturnal hypoglycaemia. This is solved by splitting the evening dose (Actrapid before tea. Insulatard at bedtime).

The woman should be seen in the clinic fortnightly to 32 weeks and then weekly to term. The insulin regime should be changed to a BD regime of a short-acting plus an intermediate-acting insulin e.g. Actrapid and Insulatard. Human insulins may be advantageous (there is a theoretical risk of antibodies to animal insulins which may cross the placenta and damage the fetal beta-cells possibly predisposing to diabetes in later life). Insulin requirements rise steadily from 12–32 weeks and fall sharply on delivery to pre-pregnancy amounts (usually about half). Urine tests are unreliable in pregnancy.

Fetal monitoring with fortnightly scans is important because macrosomia (big baby) can still occur even with good control. Monitoring with CTG traces has so far failed to predict the intrauterine deaths that can occur from 38 weeks. Fetal death has been described 12 hours after a normal CTG in a diabetic woman, therefore absent movements for more than 6–8 hours should suggest severe fetal distress.

3. *Labour* is often induced at 38 weeks because 2% of women have unexplained late intrauterine deaths. However the incidence of RDS is then increased so if diabetic control is good, pregnancy is allowed to continue to 39 weeks. Delivery is by the vaginal route but the caesarian section rate is high for diabetics (at least 20% because the obstetrician tends to opt quickly for section if there are other complications (e.g. PET, malpresentation, long labour, twins, fetal distress).

During labour and i.v. infusion of 10% Dextrose (11/12 hours) is given and an i.v. infusion of insulin is started using a syringe pump. The insulin dose (usually 0.5–2 units/hour) is titrated by hourly blood glucose measurements (aiming for 4–5.5 mmol/l). 50 units of Actrapid in 50 ml of normal saline gives 1 unit per hour at 1 ml per hour. Patients rarely need more than 2–3 units/ hour unless also having treatment for premature labour with i.v. sympathomimetics when doses of 16–20 units/hour may be needed. Hyperglycaemia must be avoided because glucose crosses the placenta, stimulating fetal islet cells and predisposing to neonatal hypoglycaemia.

Continuous CTG monitoring is performed in the usual way. A paediatrician should be present for the delivery. After delivery the i.v. insulin infusion does should be halved and the infusion continued until the next main meal when the pre-pregnancy insulin dose can be given.

4. *The baby* should be fed early (breast or bottle) and should remain with the mother. 8-hourly Dextrostix tests are performed for 48 hours to detect any hypoglycaemia.

The parents can be reassured that there is only a very small chance of the child ever developing diabetes (0.5%).

5. *Contraception*. The combined pill, POP or IUCD are all suitable methods of contraception. Sterilization is encouraged after two or three children. Only low-dose Combined Pills should be used, and because of the increased vascular risks they should only be used to delay conception for 2 years. Recurrent thrush may be a problem. There is some evidence that the IUCD has higher infection and failure rates in diabetics.

Thyroid disease   A goitre can occur in normal pregnancy because urinary iodide excretion tends to rise (like pregnancy glycosuria) causing a relative lack of iodide and hyperplasia of the thyriod (the mechanism for which is uncertain). It can be prevented by the use of iodized salt in pregnancy.

Hypothyroidism   Hypothyroidism occurs in 1% of pregnancies, and has usually already been diagnosed because it also tends to cause anovulatory infertility. In these patients the pre-pregnancy dose of thyroxine may need to be increased because of the increase in weight. However, mild hypothyroidism may present in pregnancy and is often suspected because of cold intolerance (unusual during pregnancy). It is diagnosed by a low FTI, low free thyroxine and raised TSH (specific TSH assay is best because HCG may cross-react and give falsely high TSH values), and it is treated with thyroxine (2 microgram per Kg body weight per day). Untreated the stillbirth rate doubles. Cretinism is not related to thyroid disease in the mother except in the case of rare enzyme defects.

Hyperthyroidism   Hyperthyroidism occurs in 1 in 500 pregnancies. Untreated the fetal mortality rises to 50%. Mild thyrotoxicosis is compatible with fertility. The diagnosis is suspected if there is poor weight gain or exophthalmos, especially with a family history of thyroid disease, and it is confirmed by a high free thyroxine or a positive TRH test (when TSH will fail to rise). N.B. small goitre, tachycardia, heat intolerance, palmar erythema, raised serum thyroxine and sometimes slightly elevated FTI can all occur in normal pregnancy. 95% of cases are due to Graves diseases which can be treated by subtotal thyroidectomy or carbimazole 15 mg t.d.s. Carbimazole crosses the placenta and can cause transient neonatal hypothyroidism and goitre, but no long term effects. To avoid this it can be stopped 3 weeks before delivery (half-life of 3 days) although it must be restarted because there is a risk of a post-natal exacerbation of thyrotoxicosis, and the woman must not breast feed (it is excreted in breast milk).

Neonatal thyrotoxicosis occurs in about 2% due to high levels of thyroid stimulating antibodies crossing the placenta. It can be predicted by measuring thyroid stimulating antibodies in the mother or suspected if there is a neonatal tachycardia in the last trimester. If the thyroid stimulating antibodies are known to be raised the maternal dose of carbimazole in pregnancy is kept high rather than as low as possible. Antibodies can be high even with a past history of treated Graves disease.

Neonatal thyrotoxicosis may not be apparent for several days. It causes restlessness, tachycardia, exophthalmos, goitre and feeding problems and is self limiting, lasting about 2 months. It is treated with carbimazole and propranolol and in severe cases Lugol's iodine.

In summary thyrotoxicosis in pregnancy is best referred to a specialist clinic for monitoring and control by the lowest possible dose of antithyroid drugs. A past history of thyrotoxicosis still puts the baby at slight risk of neonatal thyrotoxicosis. Antithyroid drugs are not teratogenic.

Thyroid nodule
A solitary thyroid nodule in pregnancy is difficult to diagnose because isotope scan is contraindicated. If it is solid on ultrasound scan there is a 25% risk of malignancy and if the woman is euthyroid (i.e. it is not a toxic adenoma) needle biopsy or excision are indicated.

Rare medical conditions
— Focal migraine
— Glomerulonephritis
— SLE
— Toxic erythema
— Herpes gestationis
— Acute fatty liver of pregnancy
— Autoimmune thrombocytopenic purpura
— Addison's Disease
— Sickle cell disease
— Malaria

Focal migraine
Focal migraine with alarming prodromal symptoms of hemiplegia or hemisensory change can present for the first time in pregnancy. After a few hours the onset of severe headache and nausea usually makes the diagnosis obvious. It is a benign condition in pregnancy not associated with subsequent arterial occlusion.

Glomerulonephritis
Up to 50% of women presenting with hypertension or proteinuria in pregnancy have been shown to have underlying renal disease in studies where renal biopsies have been performed. It is important to exclude this possibility because the condition can deteriorate sharply in pregnancy and occasionally precipitate renal failure. Urine microscopy provides the best test for glomerulonephritis. Increased counts of glomerular erythrocytes (of bizarre shape and size) is a sensitive and specific indicator of glomerulonephritis. Renal biopsy in pregnancy carries little risk in experienced hands.

SLE
SLE mainly affects women and its peak incidence is during the child-bearing years. If it starts in pregnancy SLE can be easily confused with pre-eclampsia, and in severe cases of PET it should be excluded by DNA binding antibody levels. SLE causes renal damage with proteinuria and sometimes hypertension, but unlike PET causes skin, joint and pleuritic symptoms and tends to worsen rather than remit after delivery. SLE can cause recurrent abortions or premature labour and PNM is increased. Self-limiting neonatal SLE can occur rarely due to antibodies crossing the placenta (rashes, haemolysis, heart-block). Patients with active SLE should defer pregnancy

until in remission. Steroid therapy throughout pregnancy is usually harmless (cleft palate, growth retardation and neonatal adrenal insufficiency are all rare). Steroid administration should be increased during labour, e.g. hydrocortisone 100 mg i.v. every 8 hours.

Toxic erythema

The commonest rash of pregnancy (1 in 120). Red, itchy, oedematous papules and plaques, starting on abdominal striae and spreading to arms and legs. Usually occurs towards the end of pregnancy. It tends to recur in subsequent pregnancies. Skin immunofluorescence is negative. It can resemble erythema multiforme.

Herpes gestationis

Rare (about 1 in 5000 pregnancies). Resembles urticarial papules and plaques, but in addition tense thick-walled blisters occur, which may be haemorrhagic. Appears at any time in pregnancy or puerperium and usually subsides within a month of delivery. Immunofluorescence shows complement deposition along the basement membrane. The infant may be born with a similar rash. Severe eruptions are treated with steroids. It tends to recur in subsequent pregnancies.

Acute fatty liver of pregnancy

This condition is very rare (1 in 10 000). The patient usually presents in late pregnancy with abdominal pain, vomiting and then jaundice, DIC and renal failure occur. Maternal mortality is 80% and PNM 70%. The patient can die within 2 days of presentation. Management is by immediate delivery with transfusion of fresh frozen plasma and awareness that hypoglycaemia can occur. It is characterized by a polymorph leucocytosis and only mildly elevated liver function tests, together with mild hypertension and proteinuria. Liver biopsy shows fatty droplets (PET shows petechiae and fibrinoid necrosis). The differential diagnosis includes:

— Cholestasis of pregnancy
— Biliary obstruction
— Hepatitis
— Severe PET
— Haemolytic uraemic syndrome
— Thrombotic thrombocytopenic purpura.

Autoimmune thrombocytopenic purpur (ATP)

Reports since 1950 on 91 patients with ATP and 138 pregnancies show a high incidence of maternal (2%), fetal (11%) and neonatal deaths (5%). It can cause haemorrhagic complications in the woman (especially intracranial haemorrhage in labour) and transplacental IgG causes neonatal thrombocytopenia in 50% of cases, which can be severe for the first week of life. The woman should ideally have a splenectomy before getting pregnant. Bleeding is likely to occur if the platelet count is persistently below $20 \times 10^9/1$. Levels above this in asymptomatic women are observed and pregnancy allowed to continue. High dose steroids and platelet infusions often fail to raise the platelet count in pregnancy. Immunoglobulin infusions may improve platelet function.

Addison's disease

In treated Addison's disease fertility is normal. The patient should already know to increase cortisol (but not fludrocortisone) intake at times of stress or fever. If vomiting occurs the patient needs 100 mg i.m. hydrocortisone as well as an anti-emetic e.g. prochlorperazine (stemetil) as a suppository (25 mg or i.m. 12.5) and urgent admission if vomiting does not settle. During labour she will need 100 mg hydrocortisone i.m. every 6 hours. She can be reassured that replacement doses of hydrocortisone and fludrocortisone are not teratogenic.

Sickle cell disease
Sickle cell trait
(Heterozygous, SA)

Occurs in 10% of Caribbean populations and 20% of West Africans. It has no effect on maternal or perinatal mortality. There is an increased incidence of urinary infections and haematuria (sickling in renal medulla). It is important to warn the anaesthetist as tissue infarcts can occur with poor hydration or inadequate oxygen levels.

Sickle cell disease
(Homozygous, SS)

Causes placental infarcts with abortion (18%), stillbirth (12%) and low birth weight babies. Pre-eclampsia, pneumonia and urinary infections are common, but maternal mortality is now negligible. Current management involves prophylactic iron (stores are often low despite classic teaching on haemolysis), Folic acid 5 mg daily, prompt treatment of infections and exchange transfusions from 28 weeks to reduce the level of haemoglobin S below 40%. Simple transfusion with diuretics can be used if the patient is already anaemic (Hb less than 7 g/dl) due to splenic sequestration. Painful sickling crises (pulmonary and bone infarcts) tend to occur in late pregnancy and are treated with analgesics and rehydration. Delivery should be vaginal. Tubal ligation should be performed on completing the family. Temporary contraception should be reliable and in Jamaica the pill or IUCD are recommended despite the theoretical risks.

Sickle C disease
(Haemoglobin, SC)

Mild and may be diagnosed for the first time in pregnancy. There are usually no complications in pregnancy but it is associated with thromboses. If the woman develops chest pain in late pregnancy or the puerperium pulmonary embolus should be assumed and urgent exchange transfusion is indicated.

N.B. Sickling tests must be carried out on all women of appropriate racial background, and if positive the husband must be checked. The infants blood must be tested by electrophoresis immediately after birth.

Malaria

Malaria in pregnancy is more severe than usual, with risks of abortion and premature labour (and rarely of transplacental transmission). Acute malaria in a pregnant woman requires speedy and complete treatment by the most effective drugs available, which are much less hazardous to mother and fetus than severe malaria.

Chemoprophylaxis is essential for a pregnant woman visiting an endemic area. Increasing resistance to the drugs together with possible side-effects on the fetus means up-to-date advice is needed on the best drug for a particular area. Chloroquine is the least harmful and usually the best choice, and will give fair protection even in resistant areas. The dose of chloroquine is 300 mg weekly (including 1 week before and 6 weeks after travelling). Congenital abnormalities do not occur at this dosage. The baby needs the usual protection from mosquito mites (nets, space sprays) because chloroquine only appears in small quantities in breast milk.

Anaemia

The importance of severe anaemia is that PNM is doubled and PPH becomes life-threatening.

Anaemia in pregnancy is defined as an Hb below 10 g/l. The red cell mass is increased by 20% in pregnancy but the plasma volume rises by about 30% therefore the Hb concentration falls due to haemodilution and the fall is more marked as pregnancy advances:

1st trimester — 12.5 g/l
2nd trimester — 11.5 g/l
term — 11.0 g/l

There is a wide individual variation in plasma volume changes. A low–normal Hb (10–11 g/l) with a normal MCV and MCH suggest the cause is simply haemodilution — monitor monthly.

The iron stores of the liver and spleen (1000 mg) should be adequate for the demands of pregnancy.

Fetus and placenta — 400 mg
Increased maternal RBCS — 200 mg
Haemorrhage — 200 mg
Lactation — 200 mg

(Also, 100 mg (9 × 11 mg) is saved by absent menstruation and in pregnancy iron absorption is increased × 2–10. Iron deficiency anaemia is becoming less common but occurs if the woman has had *heavy periods or frequently recurring pregnancies*. It is common in the tropics due to poor diet and hookworms (malaria and sickle cell anaemia lower the Hb further).

Prophylactic iron should be taken from 12 weeks to maintain iron stores, e.g. Pregaday (100 mg elemental iron as ferrous fumerate and 350 μm of folate). Iron deficiency anaemia is diagnosed by a low Hb with:

— low MCV (below 76) low MCH (below 28)

— hypochromic microcytic film
— low serum iron with a raised TIBC (diagnostic)
— low serum ferritin (reflecting low stores)

Management

1. Any severe anaemia, even in early pregnancy, needs full investigation prior to treatment.

2. Mild anaemia (Hb 9–10 g/l) is initially assumed to be due to iron deficiency and treated with 'double iron' — i.e. twice the prophylactic dosage. Hb should rise at the rate of 0.5 g/l per week. Iron should be continued for 3 months postpartum. If there is no response (reticulocytes should rise after 10 days) serum iron, TIBC and ferritin are measured and other causes are excluded:

— chronic UTI (depressed erythro-poetin; ferritin high).
— thalassaemia minor (very low MCV, Hb electrophoresis).
— megaloblastic (serum B_{12} and folate)
— continued bleeding (stools for occult blood and parasites)

Parenteral iron does not increase the rate of synthesis of haemoglobin. It is only indicated if iron deficiency anaemia (Hb less than 9 g/l) is still present at 32 weeks either due to malabsorption (no rise in serum iron measured before and after an oral iron load) or true intolerance of oral iron. Jectofer (iron sorbitol) is given by deep i.m. injection — usually 100 mg (2 ml) a day for about 7 days. It is painful and can cause headache, nausea and a metallic taste for several hours afterwards. It should not be given if the patient has a UTI (it increases pyuria).

I.v. total dose infusion using iron dextran (Imferon) is less painful. The required dose in mg is calculated thus: $4 \times$ kg body-weight $\times$ Hb deficit in g/l. Oral iron must be stopped for 2 days beforehand. Anaphylaxis can occur rarely and a test dose must be given first (with i.v. adrenaline, piriton and hydrocortisone and facilities for intubation and resuscitation to hand). It is contraindicated with a history of allergic reactions.

Transfusion is needed occasionally for severe anaemia after 36 weeks, especially if heavy blood-loss is likely at delivery (e.g. placenta praevia). All patients should have an Hb of at least 10 g/dl at the onset of labour. 1 unit of packed cells gives a rise in Hb of 1 g/dl.

Urinary tract infection

1. Urinary tract infection is more common in pregnancy because of stasis in the dilated and kinked ureters, (progesterone) increased vesico-ureteric reflux and stasis in the upper ureter, especially the right, due to pressure from the uterus in late pregnancy.

2. About 6% of pregnant women have *asymptomatic bacteriuria* ($>^5$ organisms per ml) and this is routinely screened for and treated with ampicillin, then rechecked because it recurs in 35% and:

— they have about a 30% chance of developing pyelonephritis
— if it is recurrent, there is a strong possibility that they have an underlying chronic pyelonephitis or renal tract abnormality (also said to be more likely if antibiotics fail to cure associated pyuria or if high titres of agglutinating antibodies to *E. coli* are present) and an IVU is indicated 3 months after delivery — i.e. once the ureters are a normal size again
— it possibly increases the chance of premature labour

N.B. At one time a catheter was the recognized way of obtaining a specimen for bacteriological examination. In 1955 Kass showed that an MSU (after thorough skin cleaning) with 10^5 organisms per ml had an 80% chance of indicating bladder infection, and two positive MSUs a 96% chance. The false positive rate after one MSU rises in pregnancy, therefore a positive MSU should be followed by a *catheter specimen of urine* which has a 99% chance of being correct. A single 3 g dose of a broad-spectrum antibiotic is just as effective as a 5-day course and less likely to cause thrush.

Asymptomatic bacteriuria in non-pregnant women seems to be common and transient and probably needs no treatment.

3. *Acute pyelonephritis.* 50% have had asymptomatic bacteriuria. It may present merely with nausea and malaise or with high fever, rigors, renal tenderness and dysuria. The dangers are fetal death or premature labour and permanent renal damage. Take an MSU and treat promptly with i.v. ampicillin, i.v. fluids, aspirin and tepid sponging. Anaemia commonly occurs afterwards (decreased erythropoetin). Follow up MSUs are needed throughout pregnancy.

Heart disease   1. The incidence is about 1% of pregnant women, congenital heart disease now being more common than rheumatic. The murmur may be first detected at routine examination on booking.

Mitral stenosis causes a small volume pulse, loud first sound, opening snap (which resembles a loud split second sound) and a soft rumbling mid-diastolic murmur localized to the apex.

Most *congenital heart disease* causes an obvious systolic murmur (VSD, aortic stenosis, coarctation, patent ductus). *Atrial septal defect* causes a fixed split second sound and a pulmonary flow murmur and eventually causes pulmonary hypertension.

N.B. A soft ejection murmur, oedema, slight dyspnoea and left axis deviation are normal in pregnancy.

2. Heart disease in pregnancy is not an indication for termination or elective section. Combined care with a cardiologist is necessary. With good management there should be no deterioration in the heart condition. PNM is only increased with cyanotic congenital heart disease.

3. Severe heart disease accounts for 10% of maternal mortality. Significant maternal mortality is particularly associated with

Marfan's syndrome, inoperable cyanotic congenital heart disease, primary pulmonary hypertension and congestive cardiomyopathy. Any of these conditions may be a medical indication for termination of pregnancy.

4. Pregnancy increases the blood volume by 30% and cardiac output (stroke volume × rate) by 30% from 12 weeks to term. Increased flow across a narrow valve increases the chance of LVF developing and increased rest is important — strict bedrest throughout pregnancy is necessary if LVF develops. The risk of LVF is highest just after delivery as 500 ml of blood is squeezed out of the uterus into the circulation and ergometrine (which increases diastolic BP 10–15 mmHg) should be avoided.

5. Degree of dyspnoea on exertion (to 'grade' the severity) is only a guide to behaviour in pregnancy and does not help to predict the main complications which are LVF and SBE. Increasing dyspnoea can be difficult to interpret (anaemia, hypertension, arrythmias, chest infection) and the patient needs detailed assessment.

Mitral valvotomy is rarely necessary in pregnancy but can be performed at any stage — preferably after 12 weeks to decrease the chance of miscarriage.

6. In patients with prosthetic heart valves the risk of thromboembolism is increased. If warfarin therapy is well-controlled the risks to the woman are low, but teratogenesis (6–9 weeks) can still occur and there is an increased risk of spontaneous abortion. The patient should be admitted at least 2 weeks before delivery in order to stop warfarin and start i.v. heparin before labour (heparin does not cross the placenta). Heparin is then reversed for the delivery and restarted immediately afterwards. If labour starts unexpectedly on warfarin the woman is given fresh frozen plasma and the baby Vitamin K. The risk of an abnormal baby (CNS microhaemorrhages) is less than 10%.

7. *Management* involves:

— avoid smoking and dental sepsis
— treat anaemia or infections vigorously. If fever occurs, consider SBE and take blood cultures.
— daily rest, see fortnightly, admit at 28 weeks to reassess
— digoxin, diuretics, anti-arrhythmics and warfarin are used as necessary. Plasma digoxin levels should be measured in those who fail to respond. Warfarin (fibrillation or valve prosthesis) is stopped at 37 weeks and heparin infusion started, (warfarin crosses the placenta and increases the chance of intracranial haemorrhage in the fetus).
— labour can be induced as normal for obstetric indications.
— prophylactic ampicillin is given to cover labour
— adequate pain relief is important. Any tachycardia (anaemia, infection, fibrillation, pain, fear) increases the chance of LVF developing. Epidural should be avoided if BP is already low.

— short second stage with elective forceps. Avoid ergometrine if there is a risk of LVF.

Encourage early ambulation (thromboembolism)

— discuss contraception. If LVF developed in pregnancy, sterilization is advised.

Rubella   In 1941 Gregg, an Australian opthalmologist, noticed 68 cases of congenital cataract following an epidemic of rubella, and other congenital abnormalities were soon recognised. In 1962 the virus was isolated and in 1969 the live attenuated vaccine was introduced.

Rubella antibodies are screened at booking. Girls aged 11–13 are routinely vaccinated but many are still missed. Ideally all woman should have preconception rubella screening (e.g. when prescribing the pill). A history of 'German measles' is an un-reliable guide to immune status.

If a woman of unknown immunity is in contact with rubella during the first trimester of pregnancy, take blood immediately for antibodies (IgG measured by single radial haemolysis) and repeat in 10 days (Table 6).

Table 6 Testing for rubella antibodies in pregnancy

1st test	2nd test	Action
+	unnecessary	none
−	−	immunize in puerperium
−	+	abort

If a woman already has antibodies she is immune. However if it is more than 2 weeks since the contact or if she has had a recent rubella-like illness, then the specific test (for Igm) should also be performed because a raised IgG may be due to present rather than past infection. Take throat swabs and stools for virology (within 2 days of fever or rash). If positive, abort.

The chances of congenital damage are:

— 50% at 4 weeks
— 25% at 8 weeks
— 15% at 12 weeks (deafness only)

The fetus may be stillborn or born with active infection (light-for-dates + purpura, hepatosplenomegaloy, jaundice, enceph-alitis) or have congenital abnormalities:

— cataract
— patent ductus (or ASD or PS)
— high tone deafness
— microcephaly; cerebral palsy
— micropthalmia

If the woman has no antibodies she is immunized in the

puerperium with live attenuated rubella vaccine (e.g. Cendevax or Almevax, 0.5 ml s.c.).

Breast-feeding is allowed but pregnancy is forbidden for 3 months (medroxyprogesterone 150 mg i.m. can be given simultaneously).

A mild reaction (fever, rash, lymphadenopathy, arthralgia) sometimes occurs about 9 days later.

Contraindications to this live vaccine are:

— pregnancy
— immunosuppression
— fever or infection
— thrombocytopenia (drop in platelet count following vaccination has been reported)
— allergy to neomycin, polymixin (in the vaccine)

N.B. Specific gammaglobulin during pregnancy does not help to protect the infant and is not used even if a seronegative pregnant woman has contact with rubella.

The risk of malformation after inadvertent vaccination in pregnancy is very low and it is not an indication for termination.

Infections of the fetus
— syphilis
— rubella
— CMV
— toxoplasmosis
— Herpes simplex
— Herpes varicella zoster
— HIV
— hepatitis B
— coxsackie B

1. *Virus infection*. The fetus is infected via the mother and most fetal infections are viral (except syphilis and toxoplasmosis). Cellular immunity is decreased in pregnancy and the effect of viral infections on the mother can be more severe than usual, especially polio in pregnancy. Nevertheless there is no evidence that *influenza, mumps* or *measles* specifically damage the fetus although reports of the latter in pregnancy are rare. High fever of any cause increases the risk of abortion or stillbirth.

2. *Primary CMV infection* in pregnancy can damage the fetus. It is usually symptomless (rarely it mimics glandular fever) and the only way to demonstrate an infection would be serial serology to observe seroconversion. No vaccine is available and nothing can be done to prevent infection, although known seronegative pregnant women should not nurse infants with overt CMV disease because they excrete the virus for several months. Congenital infection occurs in 1% of live births and damages about 1 in 1000. The effects on the fetus can be:

— malformations (microcephaly, retardation, deafness fits, choroiditis)

— stillbirth
— active infection (jaundice, hepatosplenomegaly, purpura)
— low birth weight
— apparently none (the majority)

In some centres women are screened for CMV antibodies and seronegative women are asked to report any fevers, so serology can be checked.

3. *Toxoplasmosis*. One third of women in GB of reproductive age are seropositive (for 1 g/G, signifying previous infection). About 0.2% of women acquire the disease during pregnancy and in about 10% of these the fetus is damaged. The infection is acquired from cat faeces or raw meat. The mother may only have a transient fever. The best method of diagnosing acute infection is by assay of the specific 1 gM by an enzyme linked immunosorbent assay. The effects on the fetus may be:

— apparently none (except positive serology)
— stillbirth
— malformation (microcephaly, retardation, fits)
— active infection (jaundice, hepatomegaly, purpura)

No live vaccine is available.

Fortunately one attack gives immunity and subsequent children are normal. Screening is possible in early pregnancy and again in 20 weeks, if negative. Women undergoing sero-conversion can be offered spiromycin (thought to reduce the risk). Perhaps all young girls should be exposed to cats to develop immunity before reaching reproductive age.

4. *Chickenpox* (Herpes varicella zoster) is rare in pregnancy because most women have had it in childhood, but when it occurs it tends to be severe. There are only eight recorded cases of fetal damage (microcephaly, fits, retardation) and only two after shingles, therefore termination is not indicated. A pregnant woman with no history of chickenpox who contacts varicella can be offered 1000 mg of specific zoster immunoglobulin within 3 days.

5. *Genital herpes*. A primary attack of genital herpes in pregnancy can cause fetal malformations (microcephaly, choroiditis) or active disease (encephalitis, hepatitis) and primary herpes in late pregnancy is an indication for delivery be section.

6. *Hepatitis*. There is no evidence that *hepatitis A or B* cause congenital abnormalities. Infection in pregnancy is not an indication for termination.

If the mother has clinical hepatitis B in late pregnancy or the puerperium, the infant is in danger of catching the infection from contact with maternal blood and should be given 500 mg specific HBsAG immunoglobulin after birth.

Symptomless carriers of HBsAG only rarely infect their baby (more common in Chinese or carriers of the e antigen).

Rhesus disease 15% of women are Rhesus negative. If the father is homozygous Rhesus positive (DD) the baby will be Rhesus positive. If he is heterozygous (Dd) there is a 50% chance that the baby is Rhesus positive. Fetal red cells can cross into the maternal circulation during delivery, abortion, APH, amniocentesis, severe trauma or external version and stimulate material antibody production (Rhesus positive transfusions will also produce antibodies). *Clinically there are two situations*:

1. *Rhesus negative women without antibodies*. Blood is taken at booking, at 28 and at 36 weeks to screen for antibodies. At delivery, cord blood is taken for blood group and Coombs test (to confirm that the cells are not coated with antibodies) and maternal blood is taken (to estimate the number of fetal cells in it by the acid elution of maternal haemaglobin — the Kleihauer test).

Usually 100 μg of Anti-D is given within 48 hours of delivery (50 μg after abortion) but a higher dose may be needed if larger numbers of fetal cells are found in maternal blood.

The Anti-D coats and destroys the fetal cells and prevents sensitization of the mother's immune system. It would be harmless (but expensive) to give Anti-D routinely to all Rhesus negative women immediately after delivery. Anti-D has to be obtained from Rhesus negative blood donors who have developed antibodies. Early unrecognized miscarriages can immunize a Rhesus negative woman and so Rhesus antibodies will continue to be seen. Anti-D is pointless and not indicated if:

a) the baby is rhesus negative
b) the mother already has antibodies

2. *With antibodies*. These pregnancies are becoming rare and are best managed in special centres. The anti-bodies are IgG and cross back to the fetus causing haemolysis with:

— anaemia
— high output cardiac failure
— oedema and ascites (hydrops)
— hepatosplenomegaly (haemopoiesis)
— jaundice (Day 1)
— kernicterus (should never occur with good management)

Fortnightly antibody estimations are performed from the time they are detected. If high (above 5 i.u.) or rising, then amniocentesis is needed to estimate the amount of bilirubin in the amniotic fluid by spectrophotometry. This is plotted against gestation on a Liley chart which is a guide to the severity of the disease. Severity is difficult to predict but tends to get worse with each pregnancy.

The severity of the disease is judged by:

— serum anti-D levels

— amniotic bilirubin levels (spectophotometric)
— scans (accumulation of ascites)

Management can involve:

— serial scans (growth and ascites)
— serial amniocentesis
— intrauterine transfusions of rhesus negative blood into the fetal abdomen (50% survive)
— maternal plasmaphoresis
— induction at 34 weeks (after L:S ratio)

Fetoscopy   Intra-uterine transfusion is not normally feasible before 23 weeks because it is technically difficult and fetal mortality is around 90%.

In a few women with high anti-D levels fetal hydrops develops before 23 weeks. In these cases direct i.v. umbilical sampling and transfusion can be undertaken as early as 18 weeks by fetoscopy. Fetal mortality is only 3–5% in skilled hands. With very high levels of maternal antibodies exchange transfusions may be undertaken until fetoscopy at 18–20 weeks. Fetoscopy can also be used to determine the fetal Rh(D) type if the father is heterozygous.

With the reduced mortality in neonatal intensive care units there is a tendency to deliver early, even at 29–30 weeks, rather than risk intrauterine transfusion.

At delivery cord blood is taken for haemoglobin, grouping, bilirubin and Coombs test (to confirm the diagnosis). Bilirubin can no longer be removed by the placenta and starts to rise immediately after delivery causing *jaundice* and the possibility of kernicterus.

Bilirubin is monitored on SCBU and *exchange transfusion* is necessary if it is rising rapidly. 'Top-up' transfusions may be needed later for anaemia.

Prevention of Rhesus   The current prophylaxis programme still fails to prevent about
immunization   700 Rh(D) negative women becoming immunized each year, because of:

— Failure to give anti-D
— Failures of anti-D to be effective
— Intrapartum immunisation

There can be no excuse for forgetting to give anti-D after abortion (therapeutic or spontaneous). Before 20 weeks gestation 50 mcg (250 I.U.) should be given, after 20 weeks 100 mcg (500 I.U.). Failure of anti-D to prevent maternal immunization occurs either because insufficient anti-D is given or because intrapartum sensitization has occurred before postpartum anti-D is indicated. The Kleihauer test (fetal cell count) estimates the size of any transplacental haemorrhage and this is particularly important after complications such as abruption, manual removal of the placenta and fulminant eclampsia (20 mcg anti-D 'neutralizes' 1 ml fetal red cells).

Giving anti-D antenatally at 28 and 34 weeks would reduce the incidence of immunization by occult transplacental bleeds. However 4× more anti-D would be needed and until monoclonal anti-D can be manufactured this would not be cost-effective using the present system of polyclonal anti-D from blood donors.

Antepartum haemorrhage (APH)

Defined as vaginal bleeding after 28 weeks (but if the fetus may be viable, i.e. from 24 weeks, the management is the same). THE CARDINAL RULE is to admit the woman and never perform a vaginal examination until ultrasound scan has excluded placenta praevia. *The possibilities are*:

— Placenta praevia
— Marginal (minor, painless) abruption
— Placental abruption
— Bleeding from the cervix (polyp, carcinoma)

1. Placenta praevia

Classically presents as recurrent painless bleeds, especially around 32 weeks as the lower segment forms. It may be unprovoked or follow intercourse. Typically the head is high and deviated to one side and does not descend onto the pelvic brim when the woman stands up. It occurs in about 1 in 200 pregnancies and is more common with twins (larger placenta). After a bleed the uterus remains soft and the fetal heart is present.

Management involves:

— Admit (Flying Squad if severe, never perform a VE)
— Resuscitate (i.v. infusion, saline or plasma expander e.g. Dextran or O-negative blood if urgent. Crossmatch blood)
— Ultrasound scan (to confirm diagnosis)
— If heavy bleeding persists — emergency section
— Usually bleeding settles. The woman is kept in hospital for the rest of the pregnancy and delivered by elective section around 38 weeks. Strict bedrest is not necessary. Blood is kept crossmatched and the fetus is monitored. Anti-D is given if the woman is Rhesus negative.

   Note that caesarian section for placenta praevia is a technically difficult operation and sometimes ends in hysterectomy to control bleeding (the lower segment does not contract down and clamp the vessels).
— A low placenta on an earlier scan — e.g. 24 weeks can rise up as the lower segment forms at 32 weeks, therefore repeat scans are indicated.

   If doubt exists an EUA can be performed at term with facilities for immediate section if the placenta is indeed covering the os. If the placenta is low but not covering the os (type 1 or 2 praevia) labour is induced by rupturing the membranes.

2. Marginal haemorrhage   Quite often a woman has a painless bleed but the ultra-sound scan shows a normally-situated placenta and speculum examination shows a normal cervix.

The bleeding is assumed to have come from the margin of the placenta. Provided it was not heavy, settles on bedrest and does not recur the woman is allowed home (after Anti-D if rhesus negative). The pregnancy is regarded as high risk because these bleeds seem to be associated with increased PNM and the fetus should be monitored for the rest of the pregnancy.

3. Placental abruption   Typically the woman has sudden abdominal pain and becomes shocked with a hard tender uterus (retroplacental blood tracts into the myometrium) and absent fetal heart. Vaginal bleeding may occur or be absent. It can follow severe trauma and is more common with severe hypertension. Proteinuria is nearly always present.

Management:

— Resuscitate: i.v. infusion, CVP line, crossmatch blood
— Morphine for pain
— If the fetal heart is still present — section
— Usually contractions have started, the head is engaged and the cervix is dilating. The membranes are ruptured, i.v. syntocinon started and delivery usually occurs without delay.
— Postpartum haemorrhage is the main risk and is often severe because the bruised uterus fails to contract properly and DIC occurs (due to placental thromboplastins, with low fibrinogen and platelets; raised FDPS)

Management involves ergometrine and syntocinon infusion (sometimes bimanual compression of the uterus is necessary) fresh blood transfusion or fresh frozen plasma. Monitor urine output, since acute renal failure can follow. Consider i.v. Mannitol (e.g. 100 ml of 25% Mannitol over 10 minutes). See the section on PPH.

Abdominal pain in pregnancy

— Abortion, ectopic
— Red degeneration of a fibroid
— Placental abruption
— Uterine rupture
— Ovarian cyst (torsion or rupture)
— Appendicitis
— Renal (pyelonephritis, colic)
— Rare (pregnancy ileus, porphyria)

1. *Pain in early pregnancy* is usually due to a threatened abortion. Pain that precedes bleeding suggests an ectopic. A retroverted uterus that fails to correct is rare but can incarcerate and cause urinary retention at about 16 weeks.

2. *In later pregnancy* the important point is whether or not the pain and tenderness is uterine. In *red degeneration* the

woman is usually over 30 and may be known to have fibroids from a previous scan. There can be fever and vomiting. If she rolls on her side the tender spot moves with the uterus. Treat with analgesics but avoid surgery.

In *abruption* the whole uterus is hard and tender, the woman is shocked and the fetal heart is usually lost. Resuscitate and induce labour.

Rupture of a uterine scar can occur silently in late pregnancy with gradually increasing pain and shock. In early labour it is suspected if pain persists between contractions. Laparotomy is necessary.

3. *Ovarian cysts* are more likely to undergo torsion during pregnancy.

4. *Appendicitis* is difficult to diagnose in pregnancy. Tenderness tends to move towards the loin from 14 weeks. Pressure in the right upper quadrant may produce pain in the RIF. There may be tenderness PR. Other 'gut' causes of pain occur rarely (peptic ulcer, cholecystitis, pancreatitis, obstruction. Crohn's disease is more common in pregnancy).

5. *Pyelonephritis* occurs more frequently in pregnancy because the ureters are dilated. Fever, loin tenderness, dysuria and pyuria usually make the diagnosis obvious. Send an urgent MSU for culture and start i.v. ampicillin. If *renal colic* is suspected, a modified IVU may be necessary (one or two exposures only). Analgesics and antispasmodics are given and surgery avoided if possible.

6. *Rare causes.* Pregnancy ileus is due to severe constipation and colonic dilation and is treated by 'drip and suck' and enemas.

Pregnancy can precipitate *porphyria* and urinary porphobilinogen should be checked if there are also psychiatric or neurological symptoms.

7. *X-rays* should be avoided in early pregnancy whenever possible. 5 rad in the first 12 weeks is associated with an 5 × increase in childhood malignancy. It is worthwhile remembering that laparotomy with ritodrine cover is much less likely to precipitate premature labour than prolonged fever and toxicity.

Hydatidiform mole

Rare: 1 in 2000 pregnancies in Britain. An abnormal cystic proliferation of the trophoblast, hence the characteristically high urinary HGC levels, hyperemesis and bilateral theca lutein cysts. *The features are*:

1. Large for dates (the uterus feels 'doughy', not cystic)
2. Vaginal bleeding ± vesicles
3. Early PET (hypertension, proteinuria)
4. High HCG (even in urine diluted × 100)
5. Snowstorm on scan
6. Thyrotoxicosis (rare; HCG resembles TSH)

Management involves 'abortion' by extraamniotic

prostaglandin followed by vacuum aspiration. Careful histology is necessary and long-term follow-up at a special centre for HCG measurements.

If HCG remains normal for 2 years the woman is assumed clear and allowed to conceive again, but needs HCG measurements after future pregnancies. Reliable contraception is needed during those 2 years (pregnancy will raise HCG levels and mask a rise due to malignancy). The Combined Pill is contraindicated because it prolongs the high HCG status.

If HCG levels rise any time after 8 weeks then chemotherapy is indicated as for choriocarcinoma.

Choriocarcinoma. About 10% of moles are malignant, but it can occur after normal pregnancies or abortions, in which case it presents as irregular bleeding, anaemia and weight loss and is diagnosed on curettings. Chest X-ray may show metastases, but early treatment with high-dose methotrexate cures 100%.

Hyperemesis gravidarum

Nausea is common in pregnancy up to 16 weeks, possibly due to high HCG levels. It perhaps serves to prevent food toxins damaging the early fetus. *Management* of persistent vomiting involves:

1. Dietary advice (e.g. dry toast before rising and avoid fatty foods) and an anti-emetic, e.g. promethazine (Avomine) 25 mg at night or t.d.s.

2. Admit if prolonged or dehydrated and ketotic. Intravenous fluids are given and serum electrolytes monitored. Prolonged vomiting can cause proteinuria, jaundice and neuropathy (due to thiamine deficiency). Sedatives and anti-emetics are less teratogenic than prolonged ketosis.

3. Always exclude a UTI. Scan to exclude twins or a mole. If vomiting persists consider other causes:

— Abdomen (appendix, obstruction, ovarian cyst)
— Raised intracranial pressure
— Metabolic (diabetes, hypercalcaemia).

4. Rarely, termination is necessary for life-threatening dehydration and ketosis.

5. In a prospective study of more than 16 000 women there was no difference in the incidence of congenital defects between those who had vomited in pregnancy and those who had not. (Klebanoff M A, Mills J L 1986. Is vomiting during pregnancy teratogenic? British Medical Journal 292: 724–6).

6. Nausea in later pregnancy can be due to reflux oesophagitis and responds to antacids.

Twins

1 in 80 pregnancies. It may be suspected if there is a family history or a history of induced ovulation with clomiphene or gonadotrophins, or excessive hyperemesis, or if PET develops in a multip.

Diagnosed by:

— large for dates
— three poles palpable
— scan (after 12 weeks)
— (X-ray at 32 weeks to exclude triplets)

THE MAIN DANGER IS PREMATURE LABOUR. Book for a unit with a SCBU. Some advocate bedrest from 28–32 weeks. Ritodrine is used before 34 weeks if premature contractions start, but if unsuccessful, section is usually performed to spare the babies the trauma of a vaginal delivery.

Strict antenatal supervision necessary to prevent anaemia or pre-eclampsia. Monitor the Hb regularly, give iron and folate supplements and admit early if hypertension occurs. Acute pyelonephritis is more common with twins. Maternal weight gain is increased by about 4 kg (e.g. 14–16 kg).

Twins are not allowed to go past 38 weeks because placental insufficiency is more common. In labour both twins are monitored (the first by scalp electrode, the second externally). Epidural is recommended because operative intervention may be needed for the second twin, which is the one most at risk.

After delivery of the first twin, it is particularly important to double-clamp the cord in the normal way in case the fetal circulations are connected by a placental anastomosis, when the second twin could exsanguinate.

Turn the lie of the second twin to longtitudinal, rupture the membranes with the next contraction, exclude cord prolapse and if necessary improve contractions with syntocinon. The second twin is at risk of hypoxia. Forceps (or traction on the legs if breech) should be used if there is any delay. Internal version (putting a hand into the uterus and pulling a leg down) is still used in this situation for cord prolapse or if the second twin remains transverse.

PPH is more likely and blood should have been crossmatched, i.v. ergometrine may be necessary.

Note: if the membrane separating the babies has only two layers (amnion but no chorion) the twins are monozygotic (identical).

Breech 25% at 30 weeks but only 3% at term. Perinatal mortality is increased (cord prolapse, intracranial haemorrhage).

Diagnosed by:

— subcostal tenderness
— balottable head
— (FH higher than usual)
— softer mass in pelvis
— VE — breech palpable through fornix (in labour identify by sacrum, anus or feet)
— ultrasound

Management

1. Observe until 36 weeks as it may well turn spontaneously
2. At 36 weeks:

— scan
— VE
— pelvimetry

Ultrasound scan excludes placenta praevia (or rarely hydrocephalus), confirms the diagnosis and measures the BPD.

VE confirms the diagnosis (which can be difficult in a primip with a deeply engaged breech) and excludes fibroids or an ovarian tumour. Clinical assessment of the size of the pelvic cavity is notoriously inaccurate.

Erect lateral pelvimetry is performed (even in multips) if vaginal delivery is being contemplated. An A–P diameter of the inlet of less than 10 cm indicates section.

3. *External cephalic version* is still sometimes attempted if a vaginal delivery is being considered.

It is performed only by a skilled obstetrician and only if the uterus is lax and the breech easily disimpacted. It should be performed gently and should be painless.

There is a risk of placental separation or cord accident. *It is contraindicated if*:

— hypertensive
— Rhesus negative
— previous APH
— uterine scar

4. *Elective section* is becoming increasingly common for breech presentations because of the higher PNM associated with vaginal breech deliveries.

Some specialists choose section for all cases, others only if there is another complication (e.g. elderly primip, bad obstetric history, borderline pelvis, pre-eclampsia, diabetic).

5. *Vaginal delivery*. Labour is induced before the pregnancy has gone past term. Epidural is indicated because forceps will be needed.

— the bitrochanteric diameter engages in the AP position and the trunk is born by lateral flexion
— Elective episiotomy
— Traction in the groins may be needed for extended legs (85%)
— If the arms become extended they are delivered by Lovset's manoeuvre (rotating a shoulder posteriorly then anteriorly again brings it down to be just under the pubic arch from where the arm can be brought down by an examining finger)
— Once the shoulders are delivered, the head is rotated to become AP (with the back upwards) and is delivered with short forceps

Unstable lie   An oblique lie is quite common before 36 weeks when the fetus is smaller. If it occurs after 36 weeks it should be corrected by version and if it recurs it is an unstable lie. The danger is premature rupture of the membranes with cord prolapse. Only if it is neglected can impacted shoulder, obstructed labour and uterine rupture occur.

Management involves:

1. Ultrasound scan. (? placenta praevia)
2. Vaginal examination (? ovarian cyst, large fibroid)
3. Admit at 38 weeks and await labour. Crossmatch blood (increasing uterine activity makes cord prolapse a possibility).
4. Some perform daily version with the rationale that a stable lie becomes more likely as the fetus gets bigger and the volume of liquor falls from about 1 litre at 36 weeks to 500 ml at term
5. If the membranes rupture, VE to exclude cord prolapse.
6. If labour starts, correct the lie. If this is not possible section is performed.
7. At term a stabilizing induction is performed. A syntocinon drip is started and the head held in the pelvis by one operator while another ruptures the membranes. Facilities for section are ready in case of cord prolapse. The patient is kept in bed until the head is well engaged.

Note: A persistent abnormal lie suggests a uterine abnormality.

Hydramnios   Amniotic fluid normally reaches a maximum volume of 1–1.5 litres at 36 weeks. It is produced from the placental amnion and fetal urine (and has the same biochemical composition as fetal urine) and is continuously being swallowed by the fetus.

Hydramnios means excessive liquor, usually from 32 weeks. It can cause pressure symptoms (dyspnoea, heart-burn, oedema or postural hypotension due to IVC compression) and is associated with a high PNM (fetal abnormality, premature labour, cord prolapse, malpresentation).

It is *diagnosed by*:

— large-for-dates
— fluid thrill
— fetal parts difficult to feel
— fetal balottement
— unstable lie

Management involves:

1. Exclude diabetes (GTT), twins (scan) and anencephaly (abdominal X-ray). Scan also excludes a large ovarian cyst.
2. If there is discomfort, consider bedrest and sedation. Repeat amniocentesis to remove fluid is possible, but it rapidly reforms.
3. Induce for severe discomfort or fetal abnormality. Prior amniocentesis can reduce the rush of fluid and the risk of

placental separation, but facilities for section should be prepared. PPH is more common.

4. Pass a firm radio-opaque catheter into the stomach of the infant after delivery to exclude oesophageal atresia.

Preterm rupture of the membranes

Left to nature, the membranes usually rupture late in labour. In about 8% of pregnancies the membranes rupture prematurely (i.e. before labour starts), and near term labour usually soon follows, or is induced.

In 2% the membranes rupture before 37 weeks (preterm). The cause is usually unknown (a few cases are due to cervical incompetence, hydramnios or trauma). *There are three problems*:

— possible cord prolapse (rare)
— ascending infection
— premature labour

Cord prolapse

In the rare event that a doctor is present when the membranes rupture, and particularly if there is a malpresentation (oblique lie or breech) a sterile VE should be performed to exclude cord prolapse.

If the cord is felt and is still pulsating (or if in doubt), replace it into the vagina (more easily done if it is wrapped in sterile gauze) and keep two fingers in the vagina, with upward pressure on the presenting part (until the woman can be delivered by section) and have someone call a Flying Squad.

Usually the woman is admitted unexamined because strict asepsis is necessary.

Diagnosis is based on the history and examination with a sterile speculum (not digitally) revealing liquor (with its characteristic odour) running from the cervix. The pool of liquid in the vagina can be confirmed as amniotic fluid with a nitrazine swab (which turns blue).

Quite commonly the diagnosis is in doubt. The woman describes an intermittent trickle but no liquor is seen.

If sterile VE reveals intact membranes, the liquor was probably coming from a *hindwater leak*, and these usually seal spontaneously. Admit for observation, monitor the fetus, and allow home after a few days if there is no more fluid.

If the problem is recurrent (? liquor ? urine) a 200 mg tablet of Pyridium is occasionally used to stain the urine red.

Management

This now tends to be conservative (i.e. admit and await events), because recent studies have shown that most neonatal deaths are due to prematurity rather than infection. Prophylactic antibiotics are not helpful, because they do not prevent infection in the neonate.

Management involves:

— admit for observation

— monitor the fetus
— crossmatch blood (in case of fetal distress and the need for emergency section)
— scan (preterm rupture of the membranes is said to be associated with fetal abnormality)
— daily HVS (some advocate penicillin if the woman is a carrier of group B haemolytic Streptococci)
— if signs of infection develop, with fever, tachycardia and discharge, the baby has to be delivered (induction or section). A raised C-reactive protein level may be a useful early indicator of infection.
— once labour starts (usually within 7 days) it is allowed to proceed. Some advocate trying to delay labour for 24 hours with ritodrine so that steroids can be given to increase fetal surfactant levels (there is no evidence that steroids increase the infection rate). The L:S ratio can be estimated on the draining amniotic fluid (provided it is not contaminated with urine), or alternatively by amniocentesis.
— before 34 weeks the baby is usually delivered by section to decrease the risk of birth trauma to the premature infant

Premature labour
1. Defined as labour before 37 weeks. It tends to recur in subsequent pregnancies. About 2% of deliveries occur before 34 weeks and with modern SCBU facilities more than 90% of babies born at 32 weeks now survive and about 50% of those born at 26 weeks.

2. Admit the woman at whatever stage to a unit with an SCBU — transfer *in utero* is safer than in an incubator. Treatment is more effective when started early so IF IN DOUBT — REFER.

3. VE to assess cervical dilatation. If the cervix is 4 cm or more, or the membranes rupture, labour is allowed to continue. Sometimes painful contractions occur without cervical dilatation.

4. Always check an MSU and treat if infected. Often no cause is found but it may be due to a UTI (which can be symptomless), high fever, twins, hydramnios, abruption or cervical incompetence.

5. After 34 weeks, labour is allowed to proceed (if gestation is in doubt L:S ratio may be indicated). Before 34 weeks, if membranes are intact, an intravenous infusion of a β-sympathomimetic is started, e.g. ritodrine (Yutopar) starting at 50 μg a minute increasing up to 400 μg per minute, (50 mg Ritodrine in 500 ml equals 100 μg/ml).

This suppresses labour in about 80% of cases if cervical dilatation is still less than 2 cm. Side-effects of tachycardia, palpitations, tremor and feelings of panic can occur.

6. If labour is not suppressed, prompt delivery is the aim, although some advocate 48 hours delay, if possible, so betamethazone 0.5 mg q.d.s. can be given to decrease the chance of RDS.

Before 33 weeks caesarian section is often performed to avoid birth trauma. For vaginal delivery, epidural is indicated (to avoid pethidine) and elective episiotomy and forceps to avoid birth trauma, with full intrapartum monitoring and a paediatrician present at the delivery.

7. Premature labour tends to recur in subsequent pregnancies. A hysterosalpingogram may be indicated if cervical incompetence is suspected, so that a cervical suture can be inserted in the next pregnancy.

During antenatal care, a digital examination can be performed at each visit to detect cervical incompetence if there is a history of terminations or premature labour.

Postmaturity   1. About 15% of pregnancies reach 42 weeks. PNM rises after this due to placental insufficiency and because the fetal head is larger and harder and moulds less easily. The incidence of fetal distress in labour is higher.

2. Why is labour delayed? The maturing fetal adrenal seems to initiate labour (and cortisol also stimulates surfactant production) and it may be that the fetus is not yet 'ready' to deliver. Sometimes gestation is not certain, when it is difficult to be sure that the pregnancy is postmature.

3. From 40 weeks the fetus can be monitored by a kick chart. Labour is not usually induced until 42 weeks unless there is another complication (e.g. hypertension). Before induction the dates should be checked and the cervix should be ripe. The fetus is monitored in labour and fetal distress in labour is an indication for section.

4. Primips induced at 42 weeks have an increased chance of failed induction or poor progress in the first stage requiring section.

Home deliveries   Between 1950 and 1980 the number of women having their baby in hospital increased in some areas from 50% to 95%. Since 1950 the PNM has fallen from 35 to 18.

There has been a recent trend back to wanting home deliveries. Some of the reasons are:

— dislike of hospital environment
— bad previous experience (self or friend)
— other children at home
— cost of travel
— statistics from other countries e.g. in the Netherlands in 1981 38% of deliveries were at home, and yet their PNM is lower than that for the UK.

A 1980 report revealed the following figures for PNM:

GP unit	6 per 1000
Consultant unit	18 per 1000
Home	23 per 1000

(Low-risk cases are selected for the GP unit). It was recommended that home deliveries be phased out further.

If a woman requests a home delivery, the GP should discuss her reasons and point out the alternatives:

— 'DOMINO' delivery, her own district midwife delivering her in the consultant unit
— 6-hour discharge
— Early transfer to GP unit nearer home

If a home delivery is planned there should be good shared antenatal care so that the consultant can assess suitability for home confinement. The community team (GP, district midwife, health visitor) must know the woman and assess the suitability of her home (heating, lighting, hygiene, additional help).

Both the midwife and GP must be present at a home delivery because mother and baby may need attention at the same time. The GP must be competent at resuscitation of the newborn and must keep his intubation technique up to date. 7% of low-risk pregnancies produce life-threatening situations (neonatal asphyxia; postpartum haemorrhage).

Planned home confinement requires strict criteria for safety. The couple must be aware of the slightly increased risk (probably 1/1000 increase in PNM) and that there is a 1 in 5 chance of needing transfer for hospital delivery for reasons detected antenatally (15%) or in labour (5%).

The woman must be carefully selected.

The following should be excluded:

— Primigravida
— Multigravida over 35, or parity above 4
— Poor home conditions
— Bad obstetric history
— Previous LBW baby
— Medical conditions (diabetes, heart disease)
— Gynaecological operations (myomectomy, cone biopsy)
— Rhesus negative
— Elevated AFP (even without NTD)

The G.P. must be competent (including neonatal intubation) and available (or have an equally competent named deputy to cover off-duty periods) and fully equipped. There must be easy access to hospital facilities and an obstetric flying squad must be available. The role of the G.P. is largely supervisory. Careful selection and monitoring of patients antenatally makes emergencies rare, but nevertheless the G.P. must be prepared.

Equipment for Home confinement (packs usually supplied by the district midwife) includes:

— Sterile packs

    — maternity pack
    — vaginal examination pack

— delivery pack
— baby pack
— repair pack

— Sphygmomanometer and thermometer
— Fetal stethoscope (sonicaid amplifier ideally)
— Entonox machine
— Amni-Hook (Hollister)
— Wrigley's forceps
— Infant Laryngoscope, tracheal tube, sucker
— Episiotomy scissors
— Sutures (catgut and silk)
— Urine testing equipment
— Blood collection equipment
— i.v. giving set. Dextrose saline
— Drugs (check expiry dates):

— Pethidine
— Naloxone
— Syntometrine
— Lignocaine (2%)
— Diazepam
— Hydralazine

Good antenatal care reduces the risks of home confinement. Routine blood tests must be performed. A routine scan at 37–8 weeks shows any placental malposition and fetal malpresentation.

The G.P. is notified at the onset of labour, and must attend early because this improves assessment later if the patients need transfer to a Consultant Unit.

Conditions indicating transfer are:

— Premature labour
— Delay in 1st stage (24h primip; 12h multip)
— Delay in 2nd stage (or failure to progress)
— Bleeding early in labour
— Fetal distress (fetal heart; meconium staining)
— Cord prolapse (1 in 2000 low risk pregnancies)

A retained placenta and PPH are indications for a flying squad. Following normal deliveries 6% of babies require assistance with breathing and the G.P. must be competent at this. Unexpected PPH or birth asphyxia are the main hazards in home confinement.

Documentation   1. Form FP24 (doctor's *claim for payment* for maternity services) must be signed by the patient at booking. Part 3 is filled in at the 6-week postnatal and sent to the F.P.C.

2. Form FW8 (*certificate of pregnancy*) must be completed by the woman, signed by the doctor (or midwife) and sent to the F.P.C. It entitles her to free prescriptions, dental treatment and milk.

3. Maternity *booking form* — filled in by the GP (or midwife) and sent to the hospital to book the delivery. If states the length of stay that the doctor or midwife feels is appropriate having visited the home. Copies are sent to:

— the maternity hospital
— district midwife
— health visitor
— GP

4. Form MatB1 (*certificate of expected confinement*) — must be signed by the GP (or midwife) at 26 weeks. The woman sends this to the DHSS to claim for maternity benefits.
5. Co-operation card — kept by the patient.

Induction of labour

1. *The indications* for induction are:

— Conditions associated with placental insufficiency, if fetal monitoring suggests chronic hypoxia (growth retardation, APH, post-maturity)
— Conditions with a known risk to the fetus (diabetes, Rhesus disease)
— Fetal death or abnormality
— Risk to the mother (PET, abruption)
— Social reasons (e.g. husband going abroad)
— It is essential to be certain of gestation before induction and if in doubt an L:S ratio should be performed first. It is a tragedy if a social induction results in a premature infant.

2. *The most effective method* of inducing labour is a combination of amniotomy and i.v. syntocinon infusion. Induction is likely to fail if the cervix is not ripe (especially in a primip) and the woman may then have to be delivered by section — if the membranes have been ruptured by more than 48 hours there is a risk of infection.

Induction is obviously contraindicated if there is disproportion (e.g. pelvic tumour, transverse lie).
3. *The cervix must be assessed.* Signs that the cervix is ripe · (i.e. favourable for induction) are:

— well-effaced (i.e. shortened)
— dilated 2 cm
— anterior (and easy to reach)
— soft
— head well-engaged (i.e. the whole of the fetal head below the level of the pubis on palpation, and on VE the head 2 cm or less above the ischial spines)

If these signs are all favourable, induction is very likely to succeed. If the cervix is unfavourable, i.e.

— long (e.g. 2 cm)
— closed (does not admit a finger)

— posterior (and difficult to palpate)
— firm

then induction is likely to fail.

The *Bishop score* is sometimes used as a guide to the ripeness of the cervix for induction. Each of the five signs is scored (0, 1, 2 or 3) and a score above 7 (maximum 13) means induction is likely to succeed.

4. If the cervix is unfavourable, prostaglandin E_2 (Prostin) in tylose gel is delivered into the posterior fornix and usually causes ripening of the cervix over 24 hours. Sometimes it even induces labour; sometimes it needs to be repeated.

A more predictable effect is obtained by placing the prostin-in-tylose extra-amniotically via a Foley catheter (pushed through the cervix and retained by its balloon — it falls out once the cervix dilates to more than 3 cm).

5. *The procedure* for induction is as follows:

— The woman should have starved overnight. An i.v. infusion is set up (in case of cord prolapse and the need for emergency section).
— Confirm the presentation
— Sterile VE to assess the cervix. Sweep the membranes and stretch the cervix (this releases prostaglandins and encourages contractions to start). Rupture the forewaters with an amniotomy hook (e.g. plastic Amnihook). Exclude cord prolapse.
— Note colour and volume of liquor. Bleeding suggests ruptured vasa praevia (blood contains HbF if fetal, HbA if maternal) and, together with fetal distress, would indicate immediate section.
— Apply a fetal scalp electrode (FSE) if possible and start continuous CTG monitoring (otherwise check the fetal heart by auscultation and apply the FSE at the next VE).
— Record the findings in the notes
— In a primip start an i.v. syntocinon infusion. (2 units per 500 ml of 5% dextrose) at 10 drops/min, doubling every 10 minutes until regular contractions occur. In a multip with a ripe cervix labour often starts soon after amniotomy; if syntocinon is used start at very low doses.

The first stage of labour   This lasts from the onset of regular painful contractions to full dilatation of the cervix (10 cm).

The woman often telephones the labour ward and is admitted if she mentions:

— regular pains (e.g. every 10 minutes)
— show (mucus plug from cervix)
— blood (usually means a show)
— 'waters gone' (ruptured membranes)

The active management of labour means that prolonged labour, with increased risks of infection and fetal hypoxia, is no longer allowed. 'No labour should last longer than 12 hours' is a working rule. The aims are:

— to monitor fetus, mother and progress
— to prevent pain and infection
— to augment labour if progress is slow

REMEMBER that as long as there is progressive cervical dilatation and the fetal condition is good, labour is normal. If abnormal then the possibilities are either augmentation with syntocinon or caesarian section.

Management includes:

1. Admit, check antenatal notes (full history if none) and examine for lie, presentation, fetal heart and the state of the cervix.
2. Crossmatch blood if:

— anaemic
— section is a possible outcome (PET, IUGR, APH, breech, unstable lie, uterine scar or previous long labour).
— PPH is more likely (high parity, twins, hydramnios, previous PPH, fibroids or if labour becomes prolonged).

3. Request an epidural (with an i.v. infusion in case of hypotension) if:

— hypertension (epidural lowers the diastolic BP)
— forceps or section is a likely outcome
— severe pain (usually a primip)

4. The woman has a bath and two Dulcolax suppositories and is encouraged to walk about in the early stages. All urine is tested. She is allowed fluids only and given 2-hourly antacid (in case urgent GA is necessary).
5. The midwife monitors (and records on partogram)

— TPR
— urinalysis (ketones, protein, glucose)
— fetal heart rate
— contractions
— cervical dilatation

6. The method of pain-relief should be considered early in labour:

— psychoprophylaxis ± drugs
— pethidine, entonox
— epidural

7. *Maternal distress* means signs of dehydration or starvation (tachycardia, oliguria, ketonuria) and is treated with 10% dextrose.

8. *Progress* is assessed by:

— cervical dilatation
— contractions (frequency, strength, duration)
— descent of the head

Cervical dilatation is slower up to about 3–4 cm (latent phase) then more rapid (active phase), but as a guide should be at least 1 cm per hour.

Contractions initially occur about every 10 minutes and steadily increase to every 2–3 minutes in established labour. The frequency of contractions is usually recorded as the number per 10 minutes (e.g. '3 in 10'), each one lasting about a minute. The strength and duration are noted as well.

Descent of the head is usually described in relation to the ischial spines, and normally the head is 2 cm above spines when it is just engaged. However, ALWAYS PALPATE ABDOMINALLY because with a lot of caput and moulding a non-engaged head can be felt well below the spines.

9. VEs must be sterile. The vulva is cleaned each time and 1% chlorhexidine (Hibitane) cream is used as a lubricant.

VE is performed on admission (and the membranes are ruptured if labour is established, i.e. with regular contractions and cervical dilatation, in order to exclude meconium-stained liquor). VE is also performed if the membranes rupture spontaneously (to exclude cord prolapse).

VEs are performed 2–4 hourly in labour to assess dilatation of the cervix and the position and descent of the head, and more frequently at the end of labour to see if the cervix is fully dilated.

At each VE *record in the notes*:

— cervix (dilatation, effacement, well or poorly applied to the fetal head)
— presentation — vertex (rarely breech, brow, face)
— position of occiput (usually LOT, then LOA then OA as it descends)
— level of head (−3, −2, −1 cm above spines, or at spines, or 1, 2, 3 cm below spines)
— membranes (intact or ruptured)
— no cord felt (cord prolapse needs emergency section if the baby is still alive)

Delay in the first stage   1. The first stage normally takes approximately 10 hours in a primip and 6 hours in a multip and 'no labour should last longer than 12 hours' is a working rule.

Active management means that if progress is too slow, labour is augmented with syntocinon because this decreases the complications of long labour (fetal hypoxia, maternal acidosis, infection).

The rate of cervical dilatation recorded on a partogram is the most important method of assessing progress (frequency of contractions and descent of the head are also important). Cervical dilatation is slower up to 3–4 cm (latent phase) then more rapid (active phase), but as a guide should be approximately 1 cm per hour in a primip.

2. If labour falls behind this sort of rate, then labour is augmented. Amniotomy is performed (if it has not been performed earlier) and i.v. syntocinon started (2 units in 500 ml of dextrose) at 5 drops/min and doubled every 10 minutes until the contractions are strong and regular (every 2–3 minutes). Good contractions will overcome minor disproportion.

N.B. Multips need much lower doses of syntocinon because uterine rupture is a possibility in a multip.

Continuous fetal monitoring is essential whenever syntocinon is used. Sytocinon is continued for an hour or two after the third stage to prevent PPH.

3. If 2–3 hours of good contractions fails to produce progress, with no further dilatation, thinning or effacement (shortening) of the cervix, then *cephalo-pelvic disproportion* is diagnosed. Often there is excessive caput and moulding of the fetal skull (and if neglected uterine rupture could occur) and section is indicated.

4. The concept of the active management of labour is largely due to O'Driscoll, who emphasizes that the most important part of good management is the certain diagnosis of labour — BEFORE any intervention to augment it.

Intrapartum monitoring   This is a screening method for fetal distress. The discovery of the relation of fetal acidosis and fetal heart rate led to fetal monitoring in the 1970s. The aim is the early diagnosis of intra-partum asphyxia. A continuous cardiotocograph (CTG) is recorded of the fetal heart-rate via a scalp electrode and of uterine contractions via an abdominal pressure transducer (or intra-uterine catheter). It is indicated in:

1. Cases where fetal distress is more likely (e.g. small-for-dates, pre-eclampsia, diabetes, post-maturity)
2. Whenever labour is induced or augmented with i.v. syntocinon
3. If the liquor is meconium stained — 10% have fetal distress (hypoxia causes gut motility and relaxation of sphincters)

The normal CTG shows:

— rate 120–160
— good beat-to-beat variation (BTBV, normally 5–10)
— accelerations (with palpation or fetal movements)

Signs of hypoxia are:

— flat trace (loss of BTBV)
— tachycardia (rate above 160)
— bradycardia (rate below 120)

— type I dips (with contractions)
— type II dips (persisting after a contraction)
— unprovoked dips (unassociated with contractions)

Combinations of these become more serious, e.g. a flat trace with a baseline tachycardia and type I dips would indicate a fetal blood sample and in some situations (e.g. early labour or trial of labour might indicate section).

Unprovoked dips in early labour usually indicate section (the fetus is unlikely to tolerate the hypoxia of strong contractions).

Type I dips are common in second stage of labour due to powerful contractions (deep ones sometimes occur if the cord is round the neck). As long as recovery is rapid after a contraction no action is needed.

The management of a poor CTG trace

1. Lie the woman on her side and give oxygen (IVC compression causes maternal hypotension). Often the trace returns to normal.

2. Exclude maternal ketosis or excessive contractions due to syntocinon.

3. Take a *fetal blood sample* — capillary blood from the fetal scalp. An abnormal CTG is a screening method and only about 50% of cases with a poor CTG trace are actually hypoxic (and acidotic).

Management depends on blood pH:

above 7.3 — normal
7.2–7.3   — repeat
below 7.2 — emergency section

Fetal monitoring is more effective than auscultation at detecting fetal distress and is the best and only method of detecting fetal distress in labour which occurs in 7 per 1000 even in the obstetrically ideal group.

Some women find the CTG bulky and intrusive. Some think it controls the baby's heart, others that it increases the chance of a caesarian (the opposite is true). Better explanation, lighter equipment, telemetry and computer-assisted interpretation will all improve acceptability.

Pain relief in labour

1. Pain in labour is due to:

— uterine ischaemia
— cervical dilatation (sacral pain)
— perineal stretching (pudendal nerve)

As the head presses on the pelvic floor, the woman reflexly pushes and this often helps relieve the pain.

2. The woman must not be left alone in labour. Understanding the events of labour decreases pain. Psycho-prophylactic techniques taught for example by the National Childbirth Trust can be very helpful (used alone or with pethidine and Entonox).

3. Early in labour, especially at night, a mild sedative is often prescribed e.g. temazepam (Normison) 20 mg.

4. *Epidural* is indicated if there is hypertension, likelihood of prolonged labour, forceps or section or severe pain (usually in a primip).

It should not be inserted until labour is established (at least 3 cm dilated with good contractions).

A needle is inserted between L1 and L2 (or into the sacral hiatus — a caudal block). The sensory fibres of the uterus go up to T11. A polythene catheter is threaded through the needle and is left in the epidural space so that repeated doses of local anaesthetic can be given, usually 0.25% bupivacaine (Marcain) about 10 ml every 2 hours. It can cause hypotension and BP must be carefully monitored after each dose. Hypotension is treated by lying the patient in the left lateral position and infusing 500 ml of Hartmann's solution. Spinal (i.e. subdural) injection can rarely cause phrenic nerve block and respiratory arrest and is therefore not practised. Analgesia is complete (although can occasionally be unilateral) and the woman also loses sensation in the legs and bladder, (examine regularly for bladder distension which prevents descent of the head and catheterize if necessary). It prevents pushing and increases the need for forceps × 10 but has no other ill-effects.

5. The alternative to epidural is to use pethidine for the first stage with Entonox for the second stage, together with pudendal block if forceps are necessary.

6. *Pethidine*. A State Registered Midwife is allowed to give 100 mg twice during labour. The usual dose is 100–150 mg i.m. followed by 50–100 mg every 2 hours up to a maximum of 400 mg in labour. It may cause nausea and metoclopramide (Maxalon) 10 mg i.m. can be given with it. Promazine (Sparine) is sometimes given as a sedative but is not analgesic and is unnecessary.

Pethidine is avoided if possible within 2 hours of delivery as it can cause respiratory depression in the newborn — reversible with naloxone (Narcan) 0.01 mg/kg.

7. *Inhalational* analgesia is often used in the second stage. Entonox (50% nitrous oxide, 50% oxygen) is used, or alternatively trichlorethylene (Trilene). It takes 20–30 seconds to be effective and needs to be started at the very beginning of a contraction. It is not used between contractions.

8. *Transcutaneous nerve stimulation*. Pain relief is based upon Melzack's Gate Theory of pain. Stimulation of large afferent 'A' nerve fibres should block smaller pain carrying 'C' fibres from transmitting to the brain. This is achieved by applying a small, variable current through electrodes placed either side of the lower thoracic and upper lumbar spine. The results have been equivocal, some women reporting benefit in the 1st stage of labour, but little or no benefit during the second stage. There have, however, been reports of an overall reduction in pethidine

needs in labour noted with its use. It seems to have no effect on the baby or the length of time of labour.

Second stage of labour   This lasts from full dilatation of the cervix (10 cm) to delivery of the baby and should not last longer than an hour. Full dilatation is suspected once the woman gets the reflex urge to bear down (as the fetal head presses on the pelvic floor). It is also suspected if

— anus pouts
— perineum bulges
— bleed (vaginal tear)
— head is visible (? caput)

It is confirmed by VE (the cervix is no longer palpable).

N.B. with a lot of caput the head may be visible before the cervix is fully dilated.

Preparations for delivery are started when the head is visible in a primip (or when reflex pushing starts in a multip). Sterile conditions are essential.

1. Rupture the membranes if still intact (rare nowadays)
2. Hold a sterile pad over the anus
3. If episiotomy is necessary infiltrate the perineum with 1% lignocaine and make the cut at the height of the contraction.
4. When delivery of the head is imminent pressure from the left hand is used to hold the head flexed and also to prevent a sudden delivery of the head (causing cranial trauma and perineal tears)
5. When the head is crowned (i.e. the occiput has passed under the pubis) the woman is told to stop pushing and pant and the head is allowed to extend slowly between contractions. The perineum is pushed down over the baby's face with the sterile pad
6. Feel for the cord round the baby's neck (30%) and slip it over the baby's head. If it is too tight cut it between two clamps.
7. Wait for external rotation of the head. Deliver the anterior shoulder with the next contraction by gently pulling the head down (towards the mother's sacrum) then upwards to deliver the posterior shoulder. If there is difficulty with the anterior shoulder (shoulder dystocia) ask the woman to push, ask an assistant to apply suprapubic pressure and if necessary put two fingers in the anterior axilla and pull down.

0.5 ml Syntometrine i.m. is given with delivery of the anterior shoulder.

8. Suck out the baby's pharynx with a mucus extractor and clamp the cord. As soon as normal breathing is established, the baby should be dried and given to the mother, who can breast-feed immediately.

Delay in the second stage   1. The head engages in the wider transverse diameter of the pelvic inlet (transverse = 13 cm AP = 11 cm). It descends onto the pelvic floor and then turns (*internal rotation*) so that the occiput turns forward and the widest diameter of the head now lies in the wider AP diameter of the outlet (AP = 13 cm, transverse = 11 cm). The head is born by extension of the baby's neck and the head then turns to the side (*external rotation*) because the shoulders remain in the AP diameter as they descend.

2. The second stage is normal if there is progressive descent of the head and the fetal condition remains good.

3. *Delay may be due to*:

— poor contractions
— poor maternal effort (pushing)
— failure of the head to rotate (OP, transverse)
— malpresentation (face, brow)
— outlet contracture (very rare)
— fetal ascites (very rare)

10% of vertex deliveries are OP.

Poor contractions in the second stage is an unusual problem now because labour is augmented at an early stage if contractions are inadequate.

The commonest cause of delay is an epidural causing anaesthesia of the pelvic floor with loss of the guttering effect of the levator ani, when the head remains in the transverse position.

4. VE is performed to determine the position. Sometimes *malpresentation*, especially brow, is not diagnosed until the second stage.

The possibilities are shown in Table 7.

5. *Management*. The second stage is not usually allowed to last longer than 1 hour in a primip or about 30 minutes in a multip (although with intrapartum monitoring if the fetal condition is good and slow descent is occurring it is safe to continue).

There may be marked caput and moulding but if the head is well engaged (examine abdominally) it will almost always be possible to deliver vaginally.

If the head has failed to rotate it may be possible to rotate the head manually to OA and then apply Neville Barnes forceps. Alternatively, Keillands forceps are used.

Episiotomy   The *indications* for episiotomy are:

— tight perineum that is causing delay in the second stage (usually a primip), or if the perineum is threatening to tear
— forceps delivery or manual rotation. In a persistent OP position (born face-to-pubes), episiotomy is usually necessary because the larger occipito-frontal diameter is distending the vulva.
— breech and premature deliveries to decrease trauma to the head
— fetal distress in the second stage

Table 7 Malpresentation

Palpation	Diagnosis	Presenting diameter and probable outcome
Posterior fontanelle (3 radiating sutures) Usually LOL then LOA then OA	Fully-flexed vertex	(Suboccipito-bregmatic) 9.5 cm Normal delivery
Anterior fontanelle (4 radiating sutures), is felt anteriorly. Sometimes the posterior fontanelle is also palpable posteriorly.	OP position, with poorly-flexed vertex (If in doubt which fontanelle is which, feel for an ear, which points to the occiput). The anterior lip of the cervix is often oedematous.	(Occipito-frontal) 11.5 cm Prolonged labour The head may eventually rotate to OA, or need to be rotated (with Keillands or manually). Occasionally the head descends OP and delivers face-to-pubes.
Anterior fontanelle and supra-orbital ridges	Brow (1 in 500) A high head may already have been noticed on abdominal examination	(Mento-vertical) 13.5 cm Obstructed labour and caesarian section
Softness (oedema) Bridge of nose, mouth	Face (1 in 300)	(Submento-bregmatic) 9.5 cm Mento-anterior will deliver. Mento-posterior obstructs and needs section.

The complications are:

1. Discomfort. Ice packs and analgesics help.
2. Haemorrhage. Vulvo-vaginal haematoma can cause severe pain and shock and needs draining and resuturing under GA.
3. Infection
4. Dyspareunia. Tight or malaligned repair which occasionally needs later surgery.
5. Recto-vaginal fistula if rectum is sutured during repair (always perform a PR at the end of the procedure)
6. Damage to the anal sphincter (and faecal incontinence) due to extension of a mid-line episiotomy

Forceps   Forceps are *indicated* in:

— delay in the second stage

— fetal distress in the second stage
— elective (prematurity, hypertension)

There are two types:

1. Low forceps (Neville Barnes) if the head is OA
2. Mid cavity rotational forceps (Keillands) if transverse or OP

The left blade is always applied first. Manual rotation (when possible) is safer than Kielland's rotation with less risk of skull fractures, intracranial haemorrhage and facial palsy. Forceps are no longer applied to a high head (i.e. above the spines) — section is much safer.

The following conditions must be fulfilled:

— head engaged
— cervix fully dilated
— membranes ruptured
— good contractions
— empty bladder (always catheterize)
— pudendal block (or epidural)
— episiotomy

The pudendal nerve curves around the ischial spine. 10 ml of lignocaine is infiltrated each side (transvaginally or percutaneously), it produces adequate vulval analgesia anteriorly but it is still necessary to infiltrate the perineum posteriorly.

Vacuum extraction

The vacuum extractor or ventouse was designed by Malmstrom and introduced into Sweden in 1954. It was used in 6–7% of deliveries in Sweden in 1983, where forceps deliveries remain rare (0.02%).

The risk of trauma to the birth canal is less but the risk of cephalohaematoma is probably increased compared to forceps. It is particularly useful if the head is in the occipito-lateral position, since the head often rotates spontaneously during vacuum extraction. The mother can still bear down and assist with the delivery.

If the fetal head is high it is contraindicated because prolonged extraction can cause fetal scalp necrosis.

Caesarian section

Ideally this is performed under epidural, with less risks to the mother and with the advantage of immediate mother-infant contact.

The rate is about 10%, and rising, due to section for fetal distress diagnosed by CTG in labour and for breech. The mortality is 1 per 1000 (which is 10 times that for a vaginal delivery) due to complications of aspiration, pulmonary embolus, haemorrhage and infection. *The recurring indications* are: cephalopelvic disproportion, two previous sections, or previous vaginal repair. The *non-recurring indications* for *elective section* are:

— placenta praevia
— pelvic cyst or fibroid
— severe PET
— placental insufficiency

Indications for *emergency section are*:

— cord prolapse
— failure to progress in the first stage
— fetal distress in the first stage
— abruption (if fetus is still alive)
— transverse lie in labour

N.B. Trial of labour may be allowed in a subsequent pregnancy following one section, but 'two sections always a section'.

The third stage   1. This lasts from delivery of the child to delivery of the placenta (usually about 10 minutes). Without intervention, there is an interval of several minutes before contractions return and cause:

a) placental separation (and bleeding)
b) placental expulsion (allowing the uterus to contract and clamp the maternal vessels feeding the placental site)

2. The third stage is now managed actively because this decreases blood-loss. Active management means:

— syntometrine (to speed separation)
— controlled cord traction (to speed expulsion)

3. Syntometrine 1 ml i.m. is given with the delivery of the anterior shoulder. Syntometrine contains 5 units of oxytocin (which acts rapidly to cause powerful contractions and speed placental separation) and 0.5 mg ergometrine (which causes sustained uterine spasm after 7 min, i.e. once the placenta is out, and lasts 1 hour).

The *signs of placental separation* are:

— fundus rises and gets harder and rounder cord lengthens
— pushing up on the uterus no longer retracts the cord
— gush of blood
— placenta visible, or palpable in the vagina

4. The placenta separates within minutes and expulsion is then hastened by controlled cord traction (the Brandt-Andrews technique).
The essential part of this technique is simultaneous upward pressure on the uterus to prevent acute inversion of the uterus (see 8 below), while steady tension is applied to the cord.
The placenta is delivered from the vagina by an up-and-down motion and blood-loss is collected and measured. The fundus is massaged to expel any clots. A syntocinon infusion (20 units

in 500 ml) is often continued for an hour or two to maintain uterine contraction.

5. *Check the placenta.* There should be three vessels (two arteries, one vein) and the presence of only two vessels suggests the baby may have renal or other abnormalities.

If the placenta is incomplete, the uterus has to be explored immediately. Inspect the membranes. A hole in the chorion to which vessels pass suggests a succenturiate lobe has been retained. If pieces of membrane are retained they pass out in 2–3 days and no action is needed.

6. Continue to monitor BP every 30 minutes, especially if there is headache, visual disturbance or epigastric pain, as postpartum eclampsia is now the commonest type.

7. *Retained placenta.* If the placenta cannot be removed, crossmatch blood and start an i.v. infusion.

It is best then to wait about 30 minutes, provided there is no bleeding, because sometimes spasm of the cervix has trapped the separated placenta and as the cervix relaxes the placenta can be drawn out.

True retained placenta is due to an adherent placenta (placenta accreta) and requires manual removal under GA (or after epidural top-up). Failure of placental separation due to uterine atony is rarely seen after syntometrine.

8. Acute inversion of the uterus causes heavy bleeding and immediate shock due to traction on the ovarian tubes. The fundus is felt in the vagina and is impalpable per abdomen. Replace immediately if possible, otherwise resuscitate and reduce hydrostatically with warm saline.

Primary postpartum haemorrhage (PPH)

Primary PPH is defined as blood loss of more than 500 ml within 24 hours of delivery. The incidence is about 1%. The causes are:

— atonic uterus
— retained placenta
— tear (vagina, cervix, uterus)
— DIC

Management

1. Resuscitate (i.v. infusion, crossmatch, and consider plasma expander such as dextran 40 while awaiting blood).

2. Atonic uterus is unusual now with routine syntometrine. It can follow long labour, hydramnios, twins or abruption and is more likely with a history of PPH.

The uterus normally contracts firmly and compresses the vessels feeding the placental site. If the uterus is not firmly contracted, rub up a contraction (which will push out any clots) and repeat ergometrine (0.5 mg i.m. or i.v.) once. A syntocinon infusion (20 units in 500 ml saline) may be needed for a few hours to maintain contraction. If the uterus fails to contract, bimanual compression may be necessary as an emergency measure (one hand on the abdomen and a fist in the anterior fornix).

3. Check that the placenta is complete. If any placenta is retained, the uterus will be unable to contract properly and manual removal under GA will be necessary.

4. If the uterus is empty and well contracted, the bleeding cannot be coming from the placental site and must be traumatic:

— episiotomy
— vaginal tear
— cervical tear
— uterine rupture (shock)

GA is essential in every case to inspect the whole genital tract. Lacerations are sutured. If bleeding continues, uterine rupture is diagnosed and laparotomy performed (haemostatic suture or hysterectomy).

5. DIC occurs rarely (usually after placental abruption), and can cause massive PPH. There is oozing from venepuncture sites and blood taken fails to clot in 10 minutes. FDPs are raised (fibrinogen may be low), and it is treated with fresh frozen plasma or fresh whole blood.

N.B. In the home the cardinal rule is to call the Flying Squad. Never transfer the patient still bleeding. Repeat ergometrine, establish an i.v. infusion if possible and maintain bimanual compression of the uterus until facilities are ready for exploration under GA.

6. PPH is particularly dangerous if the woman is already anaemic or has had a previous APH.

Acute renal failure can occur and urine output must be monitored. If this is less than 30 ml/hour correct hypovolaemia, ideally with a CVP line, and give high dose frusemide (e.g. 250 mg i.v. over 20 minutes) or Mannitol (e.g. 50 ml of 25% Mannitol over 20 minutes). If this fails to 'rescue' the tubules from necrosis, and oliguria persists, it is necessary to start the acute renal failure regime:

— restrict fluids (500 ml + output of previous day)
— high-carbohydrate low-protein diet (e.g. Hycal, 2500 kcal/ day)
— weigh daily (? fluid retention)
— monitor U and E (potassium can rise — consider 100 ml of 50% dextrose with 20 units soluble insulin in emergency. Ion-exchange resins or dialysis to remove)
— monitor urine (volume; electrolytes)
— dialyse (fluid retention, urea above 50 mmol/l, potassium above 7 mmol/l)
— await recovery, usually 1–2 weeks (polyuria)

7. Severe PPH can cause *pituitary necrosis* (rare) which can cause death or present as failure of lactation and subsequent

amenorrhoea Replacement cortisol and T4 are neccessary (Simmonds's or Sheehan's syndrome).

Maternal shock   1. The *possible mechanisms* of shock are:

— hypovolaemic (haemorrhage)
— endotoxic (septicaemia)
— cardiogenic (pulmonary embolus)
— anaphylactic (drugs, usually + bronchospasm)
— neurogenic (traction on viscera, uterine inversion)

2. In hypovolaemia decreased cardiac output causes catecholamine release with vasoconstriction to skin, kidneys, muscle (pallor, oliguria, tissue hypoxia and acidosis) in order to maintain the BP and perfusion pressure to the brain and heart.

Gram-negative septicaemia usually causes rigors and the endotoxins cause peripheral vasodilation (hence the skin is warm and red).

3. Obstetric shock is usually haemorrhagic:

— APH (placenta praevia, abruption)
— PPH (atonic uterus, retained placenta, trauma)
— uterine rupture

but if septicaemia is a possibility, take blood cultures and give high dose i.v. broadspectrum antibiotics; DIC can occur.

Management involves:

— i.v. fluids (preferably under CVP control)
— crossmatch
— oxygen 100%
— diamorphine i.v. for pain
— consider antibiotics
— consider i.v. steroids (acute adrenal failure can occur secondary to shock)
— monitor urine output (? acute renal failure)

4. *Amniotic fluid embolism* (very rare) causes sudden shock and cyanosis at the height of a contraction. CVP is raised, CXR shows mottled opacities and it is usually fatal. Postmortem reveals widespread DIC.

5. *Following GA* consider:

— aspiration (CXR; blood gases show hypoxia)
— incompatible transfusion

In incompatible transfusion, the GA masks rigors, headache and loin pain. Haemolysis and anaphylactic shock occur. Stop infusion, resuscitiate, send clotted blood (? Coombs positive, i.e. red cells coated with antibody) and collect urine (? oliguria, ? haemoglobinuria).

6. *Uterine rupture*. There are three clinical situations:

— *obstructed labour* (section should now be performed for

oblique lie or disproportion once there is failure to progress and long before the uterus ruptures)
— *ruptured scar* (the scar of a previous section can rupture in labour with sudden pain that continues between contractions and usually fetal distress — emergency section. Bleeding from the fibrous scar is often minimal.)
— *PPH* (resuscitate and laparotomy)

Bonding

Bonding between mother and infant is essential for both physical growth and emotional development. Factors that promote attachment are:

1. maternal feelings
2. physical contact
3. eye contact
4. the baby's mimicry
5. the baby's response to sound
6. the baby's crying

1. A natural anxiety about the child develops in most mothers during the early days and this promotes attachment.

Maternal feelings vary and probably depend upon the quality of mothering the woman received as a child (the incidence of battering is increased in parents who were battered themselves).

2. Close physical contact is important for bonding and a mother will automatically touch and stroke the baby. She should be allowed to hold the infant at birth.

Breast-feeding is the ideal way to promote physical contact and bonding. The baby can distinguish the smell of the mother's breast by 3 days.

Unnecessary separation must be avoided. Mother and baby should share the same room 24 hours a day. There is evidence that the separation caused by SCBU increases the incidence of battering.

3. Eye-contact is an important method of mother-infant communication. Mothers often feel particularly cut off from their child if he is blind or has his eyes covered during phototherapy.

The child can see at birth, can follow moving objects, prefers patterned stimuli and focuses best at 30 cm. Hence breast-feeding provides the ideal position for eye contact. He can recognise his mother's face by 3 weeks.

4. Mimicry of facial movements such as mouth opening or tongue protrusion can sometimes start as early as the first week. The mother feels rewarded by these copied movements, and so in effect she is being encouraged by her baby to communicate.

5. The baby can hear from birth, and from a few days responds particularly to his mother's voice. Mothers talking to their baby invariably use high pitched sounds. Analysis of film shows that the baby responds to his mother's voice by means of gestures

and movements, and that a continuous interaction is occurring between them.

6. Sound spectrography confirms that cries of hunger and pain are different and the baby uses crying to communicate demands for food attention or physical contact (cuddling). The baby thereby initiates further social interaction.

If the mother is reluctant to feed or handle her baby, or is preoccupied with her own symptoms rather than the care of the baby, these are warning signs that bonding is going to be a problem.

There may be an explanation such as a previous stillbirth or neonatal death, or it may be due to depression; the baby may be rather dull and unresponsive. Extra help from the staff can encourage normal bonding.

Breast problems
— Cracked nipples
— Engorgement
— Mastitis
— Breast abscess
— Poor supply of milk
— Drugs
— Galactocele

1. *Cracked nipples* means either a raw area or a fissure. Prevent by avoiding prolonged sucking (5–10 minutes each side is adequate); make sure the infant is taking the whole nipple and areola well into the mouth (which decreases the shearing force on the skin of the nipple) and is not repeatedly releasing the nipple due to nasal obstruction (consider 1% ephedrine nose-drops before feeds). Lanolin can be used to prevent excessive drying of the skin.

If cracked nipple occurs, rest that breast and express milk, and keep clean with antiseptic, e.g. chlorhexidine spray (Rotersept). It usually heals in 48 hours when feeding can be gradually re-introduced; if persistent, consider thrush.

2. *Breast engorgement* is common on Day 3–4, (as oestrogen levels fall, prolactin stimulates milk secretion). It is less likely to occur if the nipples are washed regularly in later pregnancy, because colostrum is secreted from 28 weeks and the ducts can get blocked.

The breasts becomes distended, hard, tender and painful and the woman is febrile.

Express milk (the electric pump is less painful than manual expression), give analgesia, support with a firm bra and avoid nipple stimulation. If severe, and breast-feeding is not desired, lactation can be suppressed with bromocriptine, 2.5 mg b.d. for 10 days (expensive).

3. *Mastitis*. Breast pain, fever, and a tender, red, wedge-shaped area on the breast. It usually follows a cracked nipple, and the baby may have an infected umbilicus. The organism is

almost always *Staph. aureus* (milk can be sent for culture).

Treat with immediate flucloxacillin 500 mg q.d.s. and analgesia. Breast-feeding can continue unless too painful. Isolate mother and infant.

4. *Breast abscess.* Mastitis worsens with brawny oedema and axillary lymphadenopathy. Stop breast feeding and suppress lactation with bromocrytine 2.5 mg b.d. Prompt surgical drainage via a radial incision is necessary, and a drainage tube is inserted.

Swab pus and continue flucloxacillin until the results of culture are known.

5. *Poor milk supply.* The stimuli for secretion of milk are:

— nipple stimulation
— breast emptying

High fluid intake is unnecessary. Feed on demand to increase suckling, and express milk at the end of each feed. If the baby is thirsty give 5% dextrose between feeds. Test-weighing before and after each feed for 24 hours often makes the mother anxious but proves whether the baby is getting sufficient milk (approximately 150 ml/kg per day). If insufficient breast-milk is available, complementary bottle feeds can be given after each breast-feed to make up the amount.

6. *Drugs.* Most drugs are only excreted in very small quantities in breast-milk. It is safe to continue breast-feeding if the mother is on warfarin, phenytoin, anti-inflammatories, bronchodilator inhalers, hypotensives, digoxin, steroids and most antibiotics (drugs should obviously be avoided if possible). Metronidazole is safe but gives the milk a bitter taste. Paracetamol is safe.

If the mother is on carbimazole, monitor the baby's thyroxine. Lithium, ^{131}I, and cytotoxics are contraindications to breast feedings. Barbiturates, benzodiazepines, ephedrine, opiates and stimulant laxatives can all harm the baby and should be avoided. Breast feeding is safe after rubella vaccination and with low dose oestrogen pills (which do not suppress lactation).

7. *Galactocele.* A non-tender retention cyst of milk that usually needs excision (to exclude carcinoma).

Puerperal fever   1. Epidemic childbed fever (puerperal sepsis) was largely due to infection with haemolytic streptococci and used to be almost as feared as labour itself.

Semmelweis observed in 1861 that it could be passed by the unwashed hands of doctors from case to case, and wrote: 'God only knows how many women I have prematurely brought down into the grave'

Temperatures above 38°C within 14 days of delivery were notifiable until recently; a midwife is still obliged to refer the patient to a doctor if the temperature is above 37.5°C for more than 3 days. *Consider:*

— genital tract infection

— UTI
— breasts (engorgement; mastitis)
— episiotomy
— superficial phlebitis (treat with aspirin)
— DVT
— chest infection (usually post-GA in a smoker)
— unrelated (influenza, tonsillitis)

2. *Examine* breasts, chest, abdomen, perineum and legs and take:

— HVS
— MSU
— blood cultures (if diagnosis uncertain)
— (throat swab)

3. The raw placental site is effectively an open wound and is predisposed to infection.
Puerperal sepsis causes fever (usually within 24 hours of delivery), foul lochia, and the uterus may be tender. The usual organisms are:

— streptococci
— coliforms
— anaerobes

Take an HVS (rigors suggest septicaemia and then blood cultures should also be taken) and start antibiotics (e.g. ampicillin and metronidazole).

Low abdominal pain and tenderness suggest pelvic peritonitis that may go on to form a pelvic abscess that needs surgical drainage.

Deep vein thrombosis (DVT)

1. The incidence of venous thrombosis is increased at least × 5 in pregnancy, and fatal thrombo-embolus is the second commonest cause of maternal death (after PET). The incidence is particularly high in women who have had a prolonged period of antenatal bedrest and are then delivered by section.

2. The increased incidence of thrombosis in pregnancy is due to:

— increased fibrinogen and Factors V, VIII, X
— decreased plasminogen activity (clots not lysed)
— venous stasis in legs (pressure from the uterus)

3. The clinical diagnosis of DVT is notoriously unreliable. Thrombosis is silent in 50% of cases and *the signs* can occur without thrombosis:

— calf pain
— calf tenderness; Homan's sign
— femoral pain and tenderness
— oedema; dilated veins
— swelling (increased circumference)

— warmth of leg
— low-grade fever

N.B. Femoral pain or tenderness are the most reliable signs.

4. Features suggestive of *pulmonary embolus* are dyspnoea (if small and scattered), pleuritic pain and haemoptysis (if moderate) or shock (if massive). Lung scan within 24 hours may show an area of decreased perfusion but pulmonary angiography is necessary for definitive diagnosis. Treatment is with heparin (or streptokinase and embolectomy if massive).

5. If the *diagnosis* of DVT is in doubt it is justifiable to wait for 24–48 hours, because the incidence of pulmonary embolus is low in DVT below the knee, and if due to other causes the symptoms may settle.

If the thrombosis seems to be extending then a *venogram* is indicated to confirm the diagnosis. Confirmation is important before subjecting the woman to prolonged anticoagulation.

Ultrasound techniques are less accurate, especially in pregnancy when the gravid uterus retards flow in the femoral veins.

Injecting *labelled fibrinogen* to label the thrombus is contraindicated in pregnancy and breast-feeding.

6. *Treatment* involves a full length elastic stocking (to improve venous flow) elevation of the leg, analgesia and anticoagulation.

I.v. heparin by infusion pump (5000 units stat. then 10 000–15 000 units 6-hourly) prevents extension of the clot. This is continued for 48–72 hours, then warfarin is continued for at least 3 months.

7. *Changing from heparin to warfarin.* Give a loading dose of warfarin (usually 30 mg) on the morning of Day 2 of heparin treatment. Stop heparin on the evening of Day 3 (so it does not interfere with the prothrombin test) and measure the prothrombin time on the morning of Day 4. According to the results the haematology lab will advise on the correct dose of warfarin (usually 1–5 mg) to be given on the evening of Day 4. Daily tests can be performed to find the correct maintenance dose of warfarin.

Warfarin therapy is *monitored by* prothrombin times (aim for 2.0–2.5 times longer than normal) or by thrombotest (aim for 5–15%; normal = 100%)

N.B. Warfarin does not increase blood loss from a well-contracted uterus. Breast feeding is perfectly safe during warfarin therapy, as only minute quantities cross into the milk.

8. *Prophylactic anticoagulation* during pregnancy is indicated if there is a past history of proven DVT.

The best method is subcutaneous heparin, 10 000 units BD (self-administered) because heparin does not cross the placenta. It decreases the incidence of recurrent thrombosis by inhibiting activated Factor X (it has no effect on prothrombin time or KPTT).

It is stopped as soon as labour starts (it has a short half-life of about 6 hours), then recommenced about 6 hours later and continued for 2 weeks.

If a woman develops a *DVT in pregnancy* it should be confirmed by venogram if possible (the fetus can be protected by a lead shield) and i.v. heparin infusion is given in the usual way, before changing to s.c. heparin.

9. *Warfarin* can be used in pregnancy — e.g. prosthetic heart valves. During the first 12 weeks it can be teratogenic (nasal hypoplasia). Between 12–37 weeks it is safe. It should be stopped at 37 weeks and changed to heparin because it crosses the placenta (and anti-coagulates the fetus, with an increased risk of intracranial haemorrhage during labour).

If premature labour occurs, clotting factors should be replenished with fresh frozen plasma.

Secondary PPH

1. *Bleeding after 24 hours and up to 6 weeks after delivery.* It usually occurs around Day 10. The lochia should gradually get lighter and any recurrence of bleeding is abnormal.

2. *The cause* is a retained piece of placenta ± infection (and only very rarely a sloughed fibroid).

3. Usually the lochia remain heavy, the uterus fails to involute and the cervix is open. With infection there is offensive lochia and fever.

4. With moderate loss it is reasonable to give ergometrine 0.5 mg t.d.s. orally for 2 days, (with analgesia because it causes painful contractions) and antibiotics (e.g. ampicillin and metronidazole). Ultrasound scan can sometimes demonstrate retained products.

5. If loss is heavy, surgical evacuation of retained products of conception (ERPOC) is necessary. Occasionally secondary PPH can be torrential and if the woman has sudden fresh bleeding (e.g. heavier than a period) she should be re-admitted immediately.

6. Early commencement of the POP often causes some breakthrough bleeding ('spotting'). If troublesome, stop the pill for a month and advise the sheath meantime.

Puerperal depression

Post-natal depression affects over 50%. These 'third day blues' consist of exhaustion, feeling weepy, mood swings, irritability, poor concentration and headaches. They last from a few hours to 7–10 days. Rising prolactin levels or falling endorphin levels are suggested causes but no causal hormonal change has been identified. About 10% go on to true depression.

Puerperal psychosis

Tearfulness around Day 3–4 is normal. Poor sleeping, rejecting the baby, distractability, multiple symptomatology or bizarre behaviour may signal impending psychosis.

The incidence of acute psychosis is increased for the 8 weeks following delivery and is about 1 in 1000. It tends to recur.

Most psychiatric hospitals have mother-and-baby units for puerperal psychosis.

The *main features of psychosis* are:

1. Changes in behaviour, mood or conversation (e.g. fragmented speech or illogical associations)
2. Feeling emotionally distant (depersonalization) or cut off from reality (derealization)
3. *Thought control* — feeling that thoughts are being put into one's mind or removed from one's mind or are known to others.
4. Feelings of passivity — feeling that one is being controlled by some external person or thing
5. *Delusions* — illogical and unshakable beliefs, e.g. 'that television programme contains secret instructions'
6. *Auditory hallucinations* — voices, usually discussing the person, e.g. 'she is disgusting, she is under my control'

If suspected, an urgent psychiatric assessment is necessary.

The postnatal examination

1. Check the following:

— Hb
— rubella status
— Rhesus — is Anti-D needed?

Hb is checked Day 5, after the postpartum diuresis has eliminated the haemodilution factor. If Hb is below 10 g/dl continue oral iron for 3 months.

If the mother is Rhesus negative (with no antibodies) and the baby is Rhesus positive, then Anti-D (usually 100 μg) is given i.m. within 72 hours of delivery.

If the woman has no rubella antibodies she is immunized, e.g. Cendevax 0.5 ml (on discharge to avoid pregnant nurses) with strict contraception (e.g. Depo-Provera) for 3 months. Breast-feeding is safe.

2. Check the charts for:

— temperature
— pulse
— blood pressure

Tachycardia suggests anaemia or infection. Following PET the BP is usually normal and proteinuria resolved by 48 hours. If not, arrange follow-up and possibly renal function tests.

3. Ask about feeding, pains (breast, abdomen, perineum, calves) and lochia (red, brown, yellow over the first week, then serous for 3–6 weeks). The recurrence of any fresh red bleeding is abnormal.

Contractions continue, especially on breast feeding (after-pains) and may require analgesia.

Perineal bruising can be painful and analgesia, ice or ultrasound can help. A dry sterile vulval pad is changed regularly to prevent infection.

Early ambulation is encouraged to prevent DVT.

4. Examine breasts, fundus, perineum and calves. The fundus involutes rapidly:

Day 1 — 24 weeks size (umbilicus)
Day 5 — 16 weeks size
Day 10 — impalpable

Slow involution can be treated with ergometrine 0.5 mg t.d.s. orally for 1–2 days (with paracetamol since painful contractions occur).

A persistent bulky uterus may be due to retained products (visible on scan) and require evacuation.

5. Note the mental state.

6. Discuss contraception, which is still necessary during breast feeding.

The POP is used instead of the combined pill if breast-feeding (oestrogens suppress lactation) and can be started on discharge.

The IUCD and the diaphragm need to be refitted at 6 weeks, after complete involution of the uterus.

Sterilization is normally delayed 3–4 months (tubes less vascular and any abnormalities of the infant are apparent).

7. Discuss any problems. The district midwife will visit the home every day for the first 10 days to check temperature, fundus, perineum, and bowels, to give advice on feeding, to ensure cord care and to perform the Guthrie test.

The health visitor visits on Day 11, to discuss future immunizations and the role of the baby clinic, and she is responsible for future developmental assessments.

The 6-week postnatal examination

The GP should visit mother and baby at least once within 7 days of delivery. The routine postnatal examination at 6 weeks has developed the reputation for being a largely unnecessary ritual. In fact, most woman like to attend and it serves several useful functions:

— symptoms (stress incontinence; dyspareunia)
— discuss anxieties
— follow-up of complications
— contraception and smear
— VE (if symptomatic)
— 6-week infant screening
— assess mother-infant bonding
— complete FP24 and register the child in the practice.

Notes

1. Pelvic floor exercises will overcome minor postpartum stress incontinence and should be explained by the doctor or physiotherapist.

Dyspareunia after episiorraphy almost always settles without the need for surgery.

2. Specific anxieties can be fully discussed, e.g. concerning

the need for future sections, or following a perinatal death or fetal abnormality — the couple may need referral for genetic counselling.

3. Specific antenatal complications may need follow-up:

— hypertension
— anaemia
— recurrent UTIs (consider IVU after 12 weeks)

4. Contraception will already have been discussed and most women will be on the pill. However the diaphragm and IUCD are not refitted unitl 6 weeks. Sterilization may be requested. A smear may be due or the date of next smear can be arranged.

5. VE is unnecessary if the woman is asymptomatic following a normal delivery. Erosion and retroversion are very common postpartum and can be ignored.

6. The *6-week assessment of the infant* normally takes 2–3 minutes; it is a useful time to discuss minor problems (e.g. skin blemishes) exclude abnormalities and reassure the mother that her baby is normal.

a) Ask about:

— birth (gestation, weight, delivery)
— sucking and feeding
— excessive sleeping or crying
— smiling (average 4–6 weeks)

N.B. Smiling in response to social overtures (i.e. when talked to) is a reassuring sign of normality.

b) Note general alertness (an important sign).
c) Examine mouth (thrush), eyes (squint, nystagmus), heart (murmur) and umbilicus (infection).
d) Ventral suspension on one hand (the baby should lift its head momentarily and extend the legs) and note any dermal sinus. Pull to sitting (head-lag should no longer be complete). Test for ankle clonus. Examine the hips (see section on CDH).
e) Growth chart. Plot weight and head circumference for birth and 6 weeks — they should both be on the same centiles. If the head is abnormally large examine fontanelles and sutures and consider referral for assessment (and possible CT scan and possible shunt).

There is a wide normal variation in development and even definitely abnormal signs can disappear. Features that IN COMBINATION may suggest some degree of mental subnormality or cerebral palsy, and indicate increased developmental surveillance are:

— prematurity or birth asphyxia
— decreased alertness, excessive sleeping
— poor sucking, irritability
— late smiling

— one limb feels stiff, hand kept closed
— movements decreased or assymmetrical
— excessive head lag, brisk knee jerks, ankle clonus

7. Assessment of maternal attitude to the baby is important. Poor bonding can lead to emotional deprivation, which causes failure to thrive.

8. Complete Part 3 of the maternity services form (FP24) and send to the FPC within 6 months to claim payment. Each of five post-natal visits (performed within 14 days of delivery) attract a fee, and the full postnatal examination at around 6 weeks attracts a further higher fee.

When the parents register the birth, the registrar gives them a pink card (FP58) to be handed in when the child is registered with the general practitioner.

Alternative methods of childbirth

The rationale for the active management of labour is that it keeps mother and baby as safe as possible. 50 years ago the maternal mortality rate was 5 per 1000 and about 1 in 20 babies died. It is now assumed that women are willing to tolerate the restrictions of a hospital delivery in the knowledge that safety is assured, as far as possible.

However, current obstetric practice is being increasingly questioned. Some women complain that having a baby involves being processed by the medical system, and that much of the routine management is unnecessary or even harmful, and spoils the enjoyment of childbirth. The medical intervention necessary for a minority of complicated labours has spilled over on to the majority of normal deliveries.

A movement for Active Birth is growing. Its aims are to support the right of women to make informed decisions about how they want to give birth, and to encourage the professionals to provide information, help and support in such a way as to further that aim.

In the quest for safety, obstetrics has evolved to become very different to the methods of childbirth seen in primitive cultures. In remote tribes in New Guinea and South Africa, for example, women squat outdoors to deliver a baby. They are support, massaged and comforted by other women. The baby is not touched until completely out of the vagina, the cord is cut but not tied, and the mother assumes immediate responsibility for the child.

The perinatal mortality in such primitive communities is around 50 per 1000. It is sometimes argued that any deviation away from our current methods might once more increase the dangers.

However, units such as that of Michel Odent in Pithiviers, France, have demonstrated that alternative methods of management can be perfectly safe. In that particular unit the emphasis is on allowing the woman freedom during labour to do as she feels.

Labour is never induced or augmented, the woman can be mobile throughout labour, and she can choose her own position for delivery (usually squatting). No drugs or epidurals are used (a warm bath is recommended for severe pain and also appears to help cervical dilatation). Forceps are not used. Vacuum extraction is occasionally used (5%). There is only a 6% episiotomy rate and a 6% caesarian section rate. The techniques of Leboyer (intended to minimize the trauma of delivery for the baby) are also used: quietness, dim lighting, delivery into water, and delayed cutting of the cord.

The perinatal mortality in 1980 was only 7 per 1000.

Routine obstetric practices are being increasingly questioned. Is the supine position, recommended for the past 300 years (and certainly easier for vaginal examinations) really the best during labour? Being mobile (so that gravity helps to dilate the cervix) and changing position frequently (with less obstruction to the IVC) would seem sensible, and some research suggests that labour is then shorter and less painful. The advent of radio-telemetry will make this possible even if fetal monitoring is necessary.

Is pethidine overused? Since 1853, when John Snow used chloroform for the delivery of Queen Victoria's eighth child, Prince Leopold, methods of pain relief in labour have received great emphasis (in Sweden all women are now entitled to a painless labour by law).

Both pethidine and epidurals restrict mobility and there are various drug-free methods of pain control that can be very effective, including focused concentration, relaxation techniques, emotional support, position changes, breath control, massage, yoga, meditation, acupressure, acupuncture and hypnosis.

It is well-known that good antenatal education and familiarity with surroundings and birth attendants helps prevent the ignorance–fear–tension–pain cycle. Should we be doing more?

Do the benefits of early amniotomy and fetal monitoring in an otherwise normal labour really outweigh the disadvantages of immobility and the risk of infection?

Is it really vital that all women in labour must starve and have i.v. dextrose for ketonuria?

Is the lithotomy position with commanded pushing really the best for delivery? Given the choice, most women prefer to squat, and there is some evidence that in this position the contractions are more effective and oxygenation of the fetus is improved.

Does an episiotomy really heal better than a large tear and cause less subsequent dyspareunia? The evidence begins to suggest that it does not.

Is a sterile field important for delivery? Would the mother touching the baby as it was born really cause infection?

Is synthometrine essential for every woman? Placental separation is also speeded by allowing the placental end of the cord to drain blood and encouraging immediate maternal suckling. Some people feel that Syntometrine increases the chances of retained membranes and delayed involution.

Should the mucus extractor be used routinely? Most babies sneeze up excess mucus and the extractor can sometimes delay the onset of respiration if used to vigorously.

Women should ideally be able to make informed decisions about how they want to have their own baby. Some women feel reassured by a fully-equipped labour ward. Others want a minimum of interference (a State Registered midwife must at least attend the delivery under the 1951 Midwives Act).

Sheila Kitzinger promotes the idea of a birth plan. Early in pregnancy (or even in the preconception clinic) the woman should have the opportunity to learn about the various options and to consider what would be most suitable for her.

To consider where she wants to have the baby. What sort of pain relief she would prefer. How much intervention she will tolerate. What the routine procedures are at the local maternity hospital. What she feels about early amniotomy and fetal monitoring. Whether she will be allowed to move around in labour and choose her delivery position. Whether she wants an episiotomy. Whether she will be separated from the baby after delivery. What will happen if complications arise and a caesarian section is necessary or the baby has to be cared for on the SCBU. How long she would like to stay in hospital.

Of course, not all women would be interested in thinking ahead in such detail, but a birth plan would help midwives to provide the personalized service that most already aim to achieve.

The ideal would be a system of care (including advanced medical technology where necessary) that is flexible enough to allow each woman to choose her own style of childbirth, that adapts to the woman's needs even as labour progresses, and that does not intrude on a couple's intimate experience of childbirth.

I am very grateful to Sheila Kitzinger, who provided helpful material for this section, and who has kindly offered to help any doctors who are interested to find out more about the Active Birth movement.

Her address is:

Sheila Kitzinger
The Manor
Standlake
Near Witney
OXFORDSHIRE

A recent WHO conference in Brazil on Appropriate Technology for Birth recommended:

— caesarian section rate below 10%

— induction rate below 10%
— no routine episiotomy
— no routine ARM
— no routine dorsal lithotomy position
— no shaving pubic hair
— no routine analgesia

The Neonate

The fetal circulation There are two *shunts* which allow blood to bypass the lungs.

1. The foramen ovale
2. The patent ductus

1. Oxygenated blood via the umbilical vein and IVC enters the right atrium and passes through the *foramen ovale* to the left side of the heart to supply the head and neck.

2. Blood returning from the head and neck in the SVC enters the right atrium from above and tends to flow into the right ventricle and pulmonary artery then through the *patent ductus* to the lower aorta, rest of the body and umbilical arteries back to the placenta.

At birth the lungs expand, pulmonary vascular resistance falls and blood is sucked from the right side of the heart and returned to the left atrium, therefore closing the foramen ovale. The Po_2 then rises and causes spasm of the ductus (prostaglandin mediated) and umbilical vessels. (Hence in RDS with a low Po_2 there is often a persistent ductus murmur). The ductus can be kept patent by giving prostaglandin E_2 (e.g. total transposition prior to surgery).

Neonatal resuscitation 7% of infants require intubation at birth, but only 50% of these can be predicted by known risk factors, (twins, diabetes, Rhesus disease, premature labour, fetal distress, breech, difficult forceps, section). This implies that intrapartum fetal monitoring should be available for all deliveries. Severe asphyxia causes cerebral palsy but the relationship between the need for resuscitation and later retardation or cerebral palsy is unknown.

The Apgar score (Table 8) is routinely assessed at 1, 5 and 10 minutes and is a numerical assessment of the baby's condition at birth. It is not particularly helpful in predicting which babies require resuscitation because this decision is only based on respiration and pulse rate and needs to be made within that first 60 seconds. The other features scored are colour, tone and grimace response to pharyngeal stimulation. Since all babies have some peripheral cyanosis, the maximum score is 9 at birth.

The procedure 1. Aspirate pharynx with a mucus extractor and give oxygen by funnel while the tongue is blue.

2. If there is no breathing by 30 seconds, use a bag and close fitting mask to inflate the lungs a few times to start off spontaneous breathing.

Table 8 Assessing condition at birth

	0	1	2
PULSE	Absent	Below 100	Above 100
RESPIRATION	Absent	Irregular	Crying
COLOUR	Pale or blue	Pink + blue extremities	Pink
TONE	Limp	Slight flexion	Active
GRIMACE	None	Grimaces	Cries

3. If not breathing by 60 seconds, intubate.

4. If heart rate falls below 100 at any time, this signifies hypoxia. Oxygenation by mask is often sufficient to restore the pulse, otherwise intubation is indicated.

5. After intubation suck out secretions with a fine catheter. Low pressure IPPV (less than 30 cm water) is used to induce reflex inspiratory movements and success is judged by a return of a normal pulse rate within 15–30 seconds.

If this does not occur, check breath sounds (unilateral if tube passed down into the right main bronchus), check cylinders and tubes, consider naloxone (0.01 mg/kg) if the mother had pethidine and order a chest X-ray (diaphragmatic hernia, pulmonary hypoplasia). Stop ventilating every 3 minutes to see if spontaneous breathing will continue.

6. Empty the stomach to prevent later aspiration.

7. Prevent hypothermia by drying the infant and switching on the radiant heater on the Resuscitaire.

8. If the baby has a bradycardia despite adequate ventilation check the pH and give bicarbonate if acidotic.

Outcome   Most babies can go to the routine postnatal ward after successful resuscitation. If it was prolonged they are observed on SCBU for several hours first. Reassure the parents.

If unsuccessful, explain to the parents, and encourage them to hold the dead infant. If staff have the courage and kindness to be with the parents and help them say goodbye to their dead child it greatly helps their later bereavement. Inform their GP.

Birth trauma

1. Intracranial haemorrhage   Torn falx due to large head or precipitate or breech delivery. The baby may either present with fits, irritability and a high-pitched cry or can be lethargic, not feeding and having apnoeic attacks. The baby is observed on SCBU, paraldehyde and phenobarbitone are used to control fits, Dextrostix and calcium are measured and an LP performed to exclude meningitis.

2. Intraventricular haemorrhage   A real-time ultrasound probe over the anterior fontanelle gives good views of the ventricular system. Research studies show

that 50% of preterm babies under 1500 g suffer spontaneous intraventicular haemorrhages in the first 3 days. They are usually small and sub-ependymal. Larger haemorrhages may be suspected clinically from apnoea, acidosis, hypotension or bulding fontanelle and be confirmed by ultrasound. If the haemorrhage extends into the ventricles it can block CSF flow and cause ventricular dilation, which if severe may need a shunt procedure.

3. Cephalohaematoma   Usually noticed by Day 3. It is subperiosteal and limited by sutures (unlike caput). Rarely it can be large and require transfusion and the absorbed blood can worsen jaundice. Even if there is an associated depressed fracture there is usually no brain damage but it can leave a hard swelling that takes months to resolve.

4. Facial palsy   Usually due to forceps and sometimes there is an area of subcutaneous fat necrosis on the face which resembles an abscess. It resolves in 2–3 weeks and meanwhile the exposed cornea must be protected with hypromellose drops.

5. Sternomastoid tumour   A lump (haematoma then fibroma) that develops in the lower part of the sternomastoid. It is associated with sternomastoid shortening and turns the head to the contralateral side. It appears around Day 7 and is gone within one year. The mother can be taught passive movements to decrease the chance of later torticollis, which otherwise develops in about 10% around the age of 5 years.

6. Shoulder injuries   Lack of spontaneous or reflex movement in one arm. X-ray to exclude fractured clavicle (no treatment) or fractured humerus which is treated by splinting the arm to the chest with a crepe bandage.

Brachial plexus injury is usually C5, C6 causing a 'waiters tip' posture (Erb's palsy). Passive movements and sometimes splints are needed to prevent contractures.

The degree of damage is always unknown but the prognosis is usually poor if signs persist after 6 months.

Ambiguous genitalia   When a baby is born the parents usually ask two questions. Is it normal? Is it a boy or a girl? The genitalia may look female but with labial fusion and an enlarged clitoris, or they may look male but with hypospadias and undescended testes. THE CARDINAL RULE is: never hazard a guess to placate the parents. Chromosomal analysis and other investigations to establish the sex take about 3 weeks but the final decision on sex of rearing may not be possible for months. It is important to defer the registration and if possible to choose a name which is suitable for either sex e.g. Julian, Francis.

There are three common possibilies.

1. *XX with congenital adrenal hyperplasia (CAH).* This is the commonest cause. All babies with ambiguous genitalia must have electrolytes monitored in case they have salt-loosing CAH. It presents around Day 3–7 as transplacental cortisone level fall. The diagnosis is confirmed by a raised pregnanetriol in urine or plasma. Lifelong treatment with cortisone is necessary, reproduction is possible and she will not be hairy.

2. *XX with partial masculinization* due to an enzyme defect in the synthetic pathway of testosterone; (one form is also salt-losing). The internal organs are male, (complete or incomplete,) and the external appearance varies from hypospadias to a little 'girl' with no vagina and inguinal lumps (testes) or herniae.

The sex chosen depends on the findings at laparotomy and on the anatomy of the external genitalia, and must be discussed with the surgeon.

Generally it is easier to construct a vagina than a penis, in which case the testes are excised and oestrogens given at puberty.

3. *Abnormal gonads (very rare).* This may be true hermaphroditism (XX or XY) with one testicle and one ovary (or bilateral ovotestes) or due to mosaicism (XX/XY). Internal organs are mixed. Again the anatomy of the external genitalia is usually the deciding factor.

Congenital abnormalities

— Spina bifida
— Congenital dislocation of the hip
— Hydrocephaly
— Microcephaly
— Cleft lip or palate
— Oesophageal atresia
— Ano-rectal anomalies
— Talipes

Spina bifida

Spina bifida occulta occurs in 10% of adult spines. In spina bifida cystica the dorsal laminae are absent and a dysplastic spinal cord protrudes through, producing a bulge on the back — a *myelo-meningocele*. (In 5% the underlying cord is normal and the bulge is just a meningocele, which can be simply repaired). The problems are:

1. 80% develop hydrocephalus due to an associated Arnold–Chiari malformation (compressing the aquaduct). It can be successfully treated by a shunt and 65% of shunted children have a normal IQ.

2. Other associated congenital abnormalities (cardiac, renal, gut).

3. *Paralysis.* With thoracic lesions the legs do not move and the child will never walk. With lumbar lesions the psoas muscles may be functioning and by transferring the psoas to extend the

hip the child may walk with full-length calipers. With low lumbar lesions transfer of the tibialis anterior may enable walking with short calipers.

4. Sensory loss predisposes to pressure sores which may require skin grafts.

5. The sacral nerves are always damaged, with urinary retention, overflow, and recurrent UTIs and hydronephrosis. An ileal conduit may be considered later in a girl. A patulous anus means there will be faecal incontinence.

If the child survives he will need repeated hospitalization and probably several operations. Early repair of the back is now undertaken in about 10% to prevent leakage of CSF and the danger of meningitis (but it will have no effect on neurological deficit).

The indications for active treatment have changed over the years. The Holter valve was introduced in 1958 and revolutionized the treatment of spina bifida. Uncritical treatment of all children however resulted in severe multisystem handicap for survivors. Babies with an adverse prognosis can be selected on day 1 and should not receive active treatment. The criteria (often called the Lorber criteria) are:

— Thoraco-lumbar lesions
— Severe paraplegia
— Gross Head enlargement
— Kyphosis
— Other severe congenital defects or birth injuries.

(For detailed discussion see Lorber J 1972 Spina Bifida Cystica. Results of Treatment of 270 consecutive cases with Criteria for Selection for the Future. Archives of Diseases in Childhood Vol 47, p 854.)

In spina bifida, hydrocephalus and anencephaly there is a 1 in 20 chance of a second affected child, 1 in 10 of a third. Screening for maternal serum AFP has reduced the incidence of neural tube defects.

Congenital dislocation of the hip

1 in 200 births.
Commoner in girls and after breech deliveries.
There is often a family history.
First the hips are abducted gently through 80°. If a hip is *already* dislocated there is resistance to abduction, then it reduces with a jolt. Next Barlow's test is performed to re-dislocate it. It is performed on one hip at a time, and with the hip flexed and slightly abducted two movements are performed simultaneously holding the greater trochanter between finger and thumb;

— push gently down towards the bed and up towards the baby's head
— internally rotate the hand 25°

The dislocated hip feels as if it is 'moving into gear' 10% of hips click, but if there is no abnormal movement it is ignored.

CDH is treated with a Von Rosen splint. This is a malleable, padded, H-shaped frame which the baby wears *under* nappies from the second day. It is checked daily at first to prevent pressure points by padding, and to check abduction is being held, then fortnightly to adjust the abduction as the baby grows (excess can cause avascular necrosis).

After 3 months most hips are normal and X-rays show a good acetabular roof. If at 12 months the femoral head is still not correctly placed, rotation osteotomy is performed.

Hydrocephalus
Diagnosed by a head circumference growing too rapidly. When hydrocephalus is likely, as in spina bifida, head circumference is measured every day. CT scan is performed to exclude sub-dural haemorrhage and a ventriculo-atrial or ventriculo-peritoneal shunt is inserted. The latter are better as they are longer and need changing less frequently and a blocked lower end requires only a minor abdominal operation.

Microcephaly
This is suspected from the infant's appearance (small forehead) and confirmed by a head circumference below the third centile. The baby is always severely mentally impaired. A CT scan is usually performed. The parents need specialist genetic coun-selling but it is necessary to exclude other causes:

— congenital infections (CMV, toxoplasma)
— craniostenosis (fused sutures needing surgery)

N.B. Rarely a reduced BPD can be due to a bicornuate uterus and this can mimic microcephaly for some weeks.

Cleft lip and palate
The lip is repaired at about 3 months and the palate at 12 months. The parents can be reassured that the results are excellent and should be shown photographs of successful repairs. A baby with a cleft palate may need to be fed by a spoon or with a specially large teat, but breast-feeding is often possible. A dental plate is fitted early to allow effective sucking. Parents should join the Cleft Lip and Palate Association. There is a 1 in 20 chance of a second affected child (1 in 10 if a parent also has it).

Oesophageal atresia
90% A blind oesophageal pouch above and a tracheo-oesophageal fistula (TOF) which joins the trachea and lower oesophagus, hence there is gas in the stomach
7% No fistula (no gas in the stomach)
3% H-fistula (but no atresia) — Cyanotic episodes on feeding and recurrent chest infections

Suspected from:

— ultrasound scan in utero

— previous hydramnios
— frothy secretions at the mouth
— cyanotic attacks
— mild abdominal distension

It should always be diagnosed before the first feed, which will cause aspiration and choking. A radio-opaque oesophageal tube is passed at birth if there was hydramnios, (in some units in all babies) and if atresia is suspected an X-ray is taken. The tube is aspirated every few minutes to keep the upper pouch clear until the infant reaches a specialised surgical unit.

Direct anastomosis is performed and the baby is fed by gastrostomy until it is healed. A secondary stricture is common and the child often needs oesophageal dilatation every few months for several years.

Ano-rectal malformations   The anus may be displaced anteriorly or may be imperforate due to:

— simple membrane
— absent anus + fistula (to vagina, urethra or skin)
— absent rectum + fistula (to vagina, urethra or skin)

Rarely there is no fistula, but intestinal obstruction. A lateral abdominal X-ray is taken with the baby inverted and a metal marker on the anus. The position of the terminal gas bubble distinguishes low (anal) and high (rectal) lesions. Swallowed air is present in the colon within 3 hours of birth.

Anal deformities can be corrected by local surgery 1 or 2 days after birth. The puborectalis ensures continence.

Rectal deformities are difficult to correct. A right transverse colostomy is performed and the definitive pull-through operation is delayed until 1 year to decrease the operative mortality. An IVU is essential because associated renal anomalies are common (also cardiac, vertebral, gut).

Talipes   Twice as common in boys. 30% are bilateral. The foot points down and the heel faces inward. If the foot can be dorsiflexed to touch the shin, it is postural due to uterine pressure. The mother is taught to dorsiflex the foot at the time of each feed and it returns to normal in 2–3 weeks.

If the foot cannot be dorsiflexed fully then the problem is structural and orthopaedic referral is necessary. Strapping is used from Day 2 to hold the foot dorsiflexed, and is replaced weekly. Severe cases may be operated on at 3–6 weeks. Otherwise, strapping continues fortnightly until the child is walking, then Denis Browne shoes are worn at night (they are joined together by a bar and hold the affected foot abducted and dorsiflexed). If these methods fail, surgery is necessary with lengthening of the Achilles tendon and division of the tight medial structures.

Talipes may be associated with neurological problems.

Examination of the newborn

The neonate is often examined the day after delivery to re-assure the parents. However examination around day 7 is also important because VSD murmurs tend to appear some time in the first week, as pulmonary pressures fall. CDH is also easier to diagnose with certainty after a few days when normal hips are less lax.

1. *Check the history* (drugs or illness in pregnancy, hydramnios, gestation and birth weight, labour and delivery, any family history of abnormalities). Most of the examination relies on careful observation.

2. *General appearance.* It is important to observe general movements, tone and reactions. Floppiness can be associated with Down's syndrome. The mother should be present as she often needs reassurance about common skin blemishes (see below). The normal baby is pale pink and often has slight peripheral cyanosis. Note any:

— pallor (anaemia ? spleen)
— plethora (polycythemia)
— jaundice
— central cyanosis (tongue, lips)
— pustules (? staphylococcal infection)

3. *Face.* Note micrognathia (the infant has to be nursed prone to prevent the tongue occluding the airway) or low-set ears (associated with renal and other abnormalities). Down's syndrome is suggested by slanted palpebral fissures, marked epicanthic folds, baggy cheeks, large, fissured tongue, flat occiput and palpable third fontanelle.

4. *Head.* Measure head circumference, palpate the anterior fontanelle for tension and assess the baby's alertness and symmetry of movements. Exclude a midline dermal sinus between the root of the nose and the occiput.

5. *Eyes.* Holding the baby up and gently swinging round usually causes the eyes to open. Exclude:

— congenital cataract
— congenital glaucoma
— coloboma
— conjunctivitis (gonococcal)

6. *Mouth.* Examine with a torch for:

— cleft palate (palpate also)
— candidiasis
— natal teeth (removed to prevent aspiration)
— cysts (gum or floor of the mouth; excised if large)

7. *Neck.* Goitre is usually obvious. The small hole of a branchial sinus, however, is ofen first spotted by the mother. Redundant skinfolds on the neck can occur in Down's syndrome

but are marked in Turner's syndrome (with widely-spaced nipples and lymphoedema of the legs).

8. *Chest.* There should be no intercostal recession and the respiration rate should be below 50/min. If these signs are abnormal, chest X-ray is indicated. Breath sounds are not helpful.

9. *Murmur*

a) A mid-systolic murmur in a well baby is usually due to a persistent ductus which closes around Day 7. Observe.

b) A loud systolic murmur or one that persists after Day 7 is usually due to VSD or pulmonary stenosis. Palpate the femoral arteries to exclude coarctation. CXR and ECG are needed.

c) A murmur with heart failure (poor feeding, tachypnoea, large liver) indicates coarctation or multiple cardiac defects (usually transposition or hypoplastic left heart) and needs urgent referral for 2D echocardiography and surgical correction where possible. (Two-dimensional echocardiography now gives very accurate information about anatomical defects.)

10. *Abdomen.* Liver, both kidneys and sometimes spleen are palpable but should not be enlarged. A palpable bladder in a boy suggests urethral valves. Examine the umbilicus for infection, discharge (persistent urachus) or herniated mesenteric duct (resembling a polyp). Inspect the anus for patency and position.

11. *Genitalia.* A hooded prepuce suggests hypospadias (refer to a plastic surgeon). Check that the testes are descended. In a girl exclude labial fusion or clitoral enlargement.

12. *Limbs and spine.* Check:

— hips for dislocation
— feet for talipes
— hands and feet for polydactyly
— spine for midline pit (above S2 it usually communicates with the theca).

These problems need referral to orthopaedic, plastic or neurosurgeon.

Harmless anomalies   Some harmless things that the mother may need reassurance about are:

1. Subjunctival haemorrhage. They disappear in 2–3 weeks.

2. Epithelial pearls (white spots) commonly occur on the hard palate. Gone in 2–3 weeks.

3. A short lingual frenulum needs no treatment and never affects the speech.

4. 'Sucking callouses' on lips. In fact these crusty folds can occur in babies who have never sucked. They can be shed and others reform.

5. Watering eye due to a blocked tear duct. This usually resolves spontaneously. If it persists beyond a year, refer to an ophthalmologist who may probe the duct.

6. Breast engorgement. Commonly occurs in male and female infants. They may lactate (witch's milk). It can last several weeks and the parents should be advised not to try and squeeze the milk out because they may well introduce infection. Spreading erythema suggests mastitis, which requires treatment with antibiotics. If an abscess forms it needs draining.

7. Umbilical hernia is common, particularly in West Indian babies and is rarely due to cretinism. It is gone by the age of 3–6 years and surgery is never needed.

8. Early urine may stain the nappies pink because it contains urates. This is harmless.

9. Small hydroceles are common. They are usually gone in 4–6 weeks and need no treatment.

10. Vaginal discharge or bleeding can occur around Day 4 due to maternal hormones that crossed the placenta. It is harmless.

Skin blemishes
1. Erythema neonatorum
2. Storkmarks
3. Erythema toxicum
4. Milia
5. Sudamina
6. Strawberry naevus
7. Mongolian blue spot
8. Port wine stain

1. *Erythema neonatorum* is a brilliant lobster-red flush that often develops all over the body. It fades within 24 hours and must not be mistaken for infection. During the first few days a line of demarcation may occur in the midline, the *harlequin colour change*, which is a harmless vasomotor phenomenon.

2. *Stork marks* (capillary haemangiomas) are present in 50% of babies, usually on the face or back of the neck. They blanch on pressure. Most fade away spontaneously.

3. *Erythema toxicum* (neonatal urticaria) is only seen in term babies and effects about 30%. It usually appears by Day 2, is gone by Day 7 and the baby remains well. It is possibly a histamine effect following contact with clothing, since it rarely affects the face, palms or soles. The lesions are red blotches, sometimes with white vesicles (eosinophils) in the middle. If these are marked with a ring it can be demonstrated that they fade after a few hours and others reform.

4. *Milia* are tiny papules ('millet seeds') on the cheeks and nose that are commonly seen in the first few days. At a first glance they often look as if some talcum powder has been left on the baby's face. They are due to blocked sebaceous ducts and fade in 1–2 weeks.

5. *Sudamina* is a rash of vesicles, usually on the forehead, that can develop in the second week. It is due to blocked sweat ducts and is more common in hot weather.

6. *Strawberry naevus* (cavernous haemangioma) is a conspicuous lesion that usually develops around 4–6 weeks. Strawberry naevi can occur anywhere, and large facial ones can be quite disfiguring. They increase in size in the first 6 months then regress, and most are completely gone by the age of 7 years. They tend to bleed easily on minor trauma, and can get infected. Parents may need a lot of reassurance that they do regress.

7. *The Mongolian blue spot* occurs in 5% of white and 90% of coloured babies. It is a grey-blue discolouration, usually in the lumbar region but sometimes over the whole back. It may be mistaken for bruising. It fades within 2 years.

8. *A port wine stain* (capillary naevus) is a developmental dilatation of capillaries, usually on the face but it can occur anywhere. It is permanent and does not blanch on pressure. In the Sturge–Weber syndrome a capillary naevus in the distribution of the first two divisions of the trigeminal nerve is associated with a vascular malformation of the underlying cerebral hemisphere that restricts its growth and becomes calcified.

Undescended testes

The testes normally descend around 36 weeks gestation. In 20% of premature male infants and in 2% of term male infants one or both testes are still undescended. *In many cases they descend during the first months, but never after a year.*

If the testicle cannot be stroked down to be 4 cm below the pubic tubercle it is maldescended. It cannot be retractile until the cremasteric reflex develops at 4–6 weeks, and then flexing the hip on that side or a warm bath will bring it down.

The child is referred to a surgeon for *orchidopexy*, usually performed at about 4 years. Spermatogenesis can be irreversibly impaired after the age of 6 and the undescended testis is 30 times more likely to undergo malignant change. 10% have an associated hernia, in which case herniotomy and orchidopexy are performed as early as possible.

Bilateral undescended testes, particularly with hypospadias, suggest that the child may be a masculinized female, and chromosomal analysis is indicated.

Circumcision

Mothers are often worried that the meatus in the foreskin is too small, and by pulling it distally the slit can be easily demonstrated. No attempt should be made to retract the foreskin until the baby is about 4 years old because of the mucosal damage which can occur, with later adhesions and the need for circumcision.

Circumcision is a religious requirement in Jews on Day 8 and in Moslems between 3 and 15 years. Even in Britain, 10% of boys are circumcised by the age of 1 year. It is contraindicated if there is hypospadias, as the prepuce is needed for repair. The only medical indications are recurrent *balanitis* or a narrow opening in the foreskin (phimosis) causing *ballooning* at the beginning of micturation.

Routine care of the newborn

1. At birth a *mucus extractor* is used to clear the nasopharynx. The soft tube can be passed down the oesophagus to exclude atresia and to aspirate amniotic fluid from the stomach, if there is meconium-stained liquor or after delivery by section. A plastic, crushing *Hollister clamp*, which does not come loose as the cord shrinks, is put on the cord about 2.5 cm from the base.

2. *Vitamin K* (1 mg Kanokion i.m.) can be given soon after birth. 1 in 400 babies develop haemorrhagic disease of the newborn because it takes the gut flora that produce vitamin K 2 weeks to get established.

Some units give vitamin K routinely; others reserve it for 'at-risk' babies, e.g. preterm, forceps or difficult delivery.

3. The baby is given straight to the mother who is encouraged to put the baby to the breast. The first bottle feed is usually 5% Dextrose and should be supervised, again in case of oesophageal atresia. The baby should be in a cot next to the mother, unless it has to go to the SCBU.

4. Immediately after birth the infant is examined for congenital abnormalities or birth trauma. Almost all serious abnormalities in neonates are apparent within 48 hours. The midwife usually assesses the Apgar score at 1, 5 and 10 minutes, weighs the baby, measures its length and head circumference, takes a rectal temperature, puts a plastic identification band on the wrist and checks that there are three placental vessels (two suggests a renal anomaly).

5. The full routine examination of the neonate is performed by the houseman the day after delivery or before discharge. The mother should be present so she can discuss any problems (see skin blemishes and harmless anomalies). If an abnormality is found, a nurse should be present when the mother is told, so they can discuss it later.

6. Vernix is wiped off the baby's face at birth but otherwise this is left to flake off. The baby is *bathed* once on the day of discharge. The normal newborn sleeps most of the time between feeds, crying only if hungry, thirsty or in pain.

7. *Dextrostix* are important 8-hourly for 48 hours if the baby is liable to hypoglycaemia (i.e. is small-for-dates or the mother was diabetic). Significant hypoglycaemia in a neonate is a level below 1 mmol/l (20 mg/dl).

8. *The cord* is kept dry and clean with chlorhexidine in spirit daily. It usually separates around Day 7 and then takes 3–4 days to granulate over. It must be inspected daily for signs of infection, and this is one reason why the district midwife visits daily after discharge.

9. The midwife charts the weight and temperature and inspects skin, eyes, mouth (for thrush) and umbilicus daily. The rectal temperature should not drop below 36°C. Weight loss occurs for the first 4 days and birth weight is regained by about Day 10. Eye drops or swabs are no longer used routinely. Regular observation is important and any discharge is swabbed for culture. Gonococcal conjunctivitis can blind and is notifiable. It is treated with neomycin eye drops and systemic penicillin.

10. *Urine* is often passed soon after delivery and may be dark or pink at first. Pressure on the bladder may stimulate micturition, but no urine by 24 hours suggests urethral valves. Sticky, dark green *meconium* is normally passed within a few hours of delivery and is often preceded by a white plug of mucus. No meconium by 48 hours suggests intestinal obstruction. The stools become more liquid and yellow after 3 or 4 days of milk.

11. The *Guthrie test* is routinely performed on Day 7, after 6 days of milk feeds. Capillary blood is taken from a heel prick and tested for phenylalanine and if high, due to phenylketonuria, a low phenylalanine diet can prevent brain damage. All areas now screen for TSH on the same sample to detect hypothyroidism.

Nappy rash
— Ammoniacal dermatitis
— Seborrhoeic dermatitis
— Frequent loose stools
— Candidiasis
— Contact sensitivity (washing powder)

1. *Ammoniacal dermatitis* is due to continually damp nappies (faecal bacteria break down the urea to produce ammonia). Erythema and erosion appear. It soon heals if left exposed. Otherwise, advise changing napkins regularly, using napkin liners and applying a protective cream (zinc or silicone) at each change. If it has not healed within a week there is usually a secondary infection with *Candida*, or a contact sensitivity (rinse nappies thoroughly).

2. *Seborrhoeic dermatitis* always begins before the age of 3 months and is gone by 9 months. It is a badly-named rash characterised by erythema and scaling in the napkin area and also affecting the neck, face and scalp (cradle cap). There is no itching or soreness. The baby remains characteristically well. The rash clears within a few weeks with 1% hydrocortisone. Crusts on the scalp can be removed with 0.5% salicylic acid in soft paraffin, left on the scalp for an hour, then removed with shampoo. Again, secondary infection with bacteria or *Candida* is common.

3. *Peri-anal excoriation* is usually due to diarrhoea and frequent acid stools. Expose and protect with zinc cream.

4. *Candidiasis* is fiery red with a scaly margin and satellite

lesions. Treat with nystatin cream at every nappy change. Check for *Candida* in the baby's mouth or the mother's breast.

Bottle-feeding

1. There is little to choose between the various brands of milk for normal babies, and the common habit of running the gamut to find the one which suits the baby is illogical. Cow's milk preparations are 'humanized' and mimic human milk by being low in protein, high in lactose and low in solute. They are fortified with vitamins and iron.

2. Hospitals now use pre-packed sterilized feeds. Once at home the mother has to learn how to measure out scoops of a dried powder formula, and mistakes are common. The bottle and teats should be kept in dilute hypochlorite (Milton). If bottles are made up early they should be kept in the fridge and re-warmed before use. Undiluted cow's milk (doorstep milk) is too concentrated, and should not be used before 6 months (and should be boiled then cooled before 12 months).

3. The first feed is given as early as possible after birth.

4. The baby needs 150 ml per kg/day (2½ oz/lb per day). The amount given is increased (to mimic breast-feeding) from 20 ml/kg on Day 1 to 40 ml/kg on Day 2 etc, so 150 ml/kg is reached by Day 7.

N.B. 1 oz = 30 ml = 30 gm is a useful equation when discussing feeds with non-metric mothers.

5. The baby is fed every 3–4 hours at first, missing out the night feed after a few weeks. This regime should be flexible, because all babies are different, 150 ml/kg per day is a guide, and the baby can usually be fed to satisfy its appetite. A baby that is crying may be thirsty rather than hungry. Premature babies need relatively more, e.g. 200 ml/kg per day.

6. *Allergy* to cow's milk protein can occur, causing diarrhoea and colic. They may be a family history of atopy. The baby may have a peri-oral rash. Experimentally, blood mixed with milk produces high levels of histamine. The baby can be fed on a soya-based milk (e.g. Wysoy, Formula S).

Breast-feeding

Compared to cow's milk, human milk has:

1. *More lactose*, and therefore (since human milk is isosmolar) less solute. This makes the gut contents more acidic and hence more bactericidal.

2. *Less protein*, and a ratio of casein to lactalbumin of 1:1 (cow's milk is 4:1), making it more easily absorbed.

3. *The same quantity of fat*, but with a higher level of poly-unsaturated fats, which are possibly essential, and the fat is more easily absorbed.

4. Possible *bactericidal factors*: IgA, lysozyme, lymphocytes, lactoferrin and prostaglandins. The gut contents of breast-fed babies are virtually sterile and they never get gastroenteritis. The first colostrum is particularly rich in IgA.

Advantages 1. It is the ideal way to promote bonding.

2. The fat and protein content are ideal and better absorbed (and possibly vary as the child grows). Obesity is rarely a problem in breast-fed babies.

3. Suckling stimulates oxytocin release and speeds up involution of the uterus (the after-pains of feeding).

4. No danger of gastroenteritis.

5. Less danger of cow's milk protein allergy (and possibly eczema). For this reason, if complimentary feeds are necessary, a pre-digested milk can be used (e.g. Progestamilk).

6. Problems that used to be associated with bottle-feeding were obesity, hypernatraemia and hypocalcaemia (high phosphates binding calcium), but these are now uncommon with the low-solute humanized preparations.

Physiology 1. Colostrum appears from 28 weeks; consequently the nipples should be washed regularly in later pregnancy because blocked lactiferous ducts predispose to later breast engorgement.

2. The high levels of oestrogen in pregnancy inhibit prolactin secretion, but as these fall, milk secretion starts, hence engorgement tends to occur around Day 4. Nipple stimulation also causes prolactin secretion.

3. Suckling causes oxytocin release and contraction of the myo-epithelial cells (and uterus) and milk let-down. This reflex is strongly influenced by higher centres, and the baby's cry can cause milk let-down. Conversely, if the mother feels anxious or nervous, milk let-down can be completely inhibited.

Spurts of milk can occur, due to this reflex, and this does not mean that there is necessarily a lot of milk available.

4. The *best stimuli for milk production* are:

— frequent suckling
— breast emptying

Therefore, if there is insufficient milk the baby should be put to the breast more frequently and the breasts should be expressed after each feed to ensure they are completely empty.

A high fluid intake is totally unnecessary — starving mothers can produce adequate breast-milk. Each breast produces about 50 ml per feed.

General advice 1. Start breast-feeding in the labour ward. Babies are often reluctant to take the nipple at first and the mother may need encouragement to persist. The baby should have its neck slightly extended and the whole nipple well inside its mouth.

2. Build up with 3, 5, 7, then 10 minutes on each breast and wind between sides. In fact, most of the milk is taken within the first 5 minutes.

3. Demand feeding helps bonding and improves milk-flow.

4. Express the breasts after each feed to improve milk flow.

5. Colostrum is secreted for 2 days, then milk starts to appear. If the baby is hungry, encourage suckling. Give 5% dextrose before resorting to complementary milk feeds. A well-hydrated baby can manage on little milk, certainly for the first 5 days.

6. The stools in breast-fed babies can be green and very frequent (e.g. hourly) when abundant milk starts to flow around Day 5, but characteristically they become less frequent, and by a month may only occur every few days (one more advantage of breast-feeding!).

7. It is advised to give breast-fed babies 7 drops per day of NHS 'A and D drops' until the age of 1 year.

Feeding problems

1. *Poor weight gain.* The baby loses weight for about 4 days, regains its birthweight by about Day 10 and then gains about 30 g a day for the first 4 months ('an ounce a day except on Sundays').

Plotting a growth chart is the best way to assess adequate intake, but as a guide the baby should double his birthweight by 5 months. If growth is poor he needs larger and more frequent feeds.

2. *Air swallowing* can cause possetting (regurgitating milk) and may be due to the hole in the teat being too small or too large. Troublesome regurgitation can sometimes be reduced by thickening the feeds.

Sometimes gulping occurs if breast-milk let-down is rapid, especially on the first feed of the day. Adequate winding is advised, and if this problem is very troublesome, the first 30 ml can be expressed and refed later.

3. *Hunger.* The baby may seem continually hungry. He may just be thirsty, especially in hot weather, and need extra water rather than milk. He may indeed not be getting enough milk, and the mother's method of making up feeds should be checked. He may just be greedy, and as a last resort 30 mg chloral hydrate before alternate feeds can be tried for a week.

4. *Insufficient milk.* Breast-fed babies can sometimes get insufficient milk without complaining, and they can develop dark green stools with mucus (starvation stools).

The amount of breast-milk the baby is getting can be worked out by test-weighing him before and after each feed, and if increased suckling and expressing does not increase the supply, complementary feeds or a change to bottle-feeding may be necessary.

Test-weighing has to be carried out over 24 hours to be accurate, and often causes maternal anxiety.

5. *Cracked nipples, engorgement, mastitis, breast abscess and drugs* are dealt with in the section on the breast.

6. *Reluctance to feed* may be due to oral thrush or a blocked nose, but can be a sign of severe illness.

The low-birth-weight baby

About 70% of all babies weigh 2.5 kg or less at birth and are defined as low birth weight (LBW). About two thirds of these are preterm and one third are small-for-dates.

90% of LBW babies spend some time in SCBU and babies under 1.5 kg may spend 3 or more months there. Babies under 750 g or of less than 26 weeks gestation are unlikely to survive.

Neonatal intensive care may involve:

— biochemical monitoring
— umbilical artery catheterization (for gases)
— mechanical ventilation
— total parenteral feeding
— drug therapy (mainly antibiotics)

Vitamin supplements (e.g. Abidec 0.6 ml daily) are given from the second week to the age of 2. Iron supplements are started once the baby is 6 weeks and continued for 6 months.

Regional SCBUs have definitely lowered the mortality rate (by about 2 per 1000). There has also been a dramatic reduction in cerebral palsy (diplegia, hemiplegia and quadriplegia) in LBW babies. However, long-term follow-up studies of LBW babies that survive the SCBU are needed. Preliminary reports suggest that poor bonding, slow development and clumsiness are more common.

The pre-term infant

1. The pre-term infant is defined as a baby of less than 37 weeks gestation. More than 90% of those born at 32 weeks now survive. About 50% of those born at 26 weeks (about 800 g) should now survive, and regional SCBU results will be even better. The cause for premature labour is usually unknown. Compared with the SFD baby, the pre-term is less at risk during labour and delivery but is *especially vulnerable during the neonatal period due to immaturity of organ systems.*

2. The baby has a feeble cry and a characteristic appearance with thin, red, shiny skin, lanugo, no vernix, relatively large head, a protuberant abdomen and a frog position of the legs due to poor tone. The clitoris appears large and intersex may be suspected, mistakenly. The testes may be undescended.

3. The baby has poor temperature regulation, poor sucking, swallowing and breathing reflexes and a tendency to apnoeic attacks. It therefore needs to be nursed in an incubator on an apnoea mattress, and tube-fed via a nasogastric tube. The other problems are:

— RDS (occurs in 50% under 32 weeks)
— jaundice (immature liver enzymes systems)
— intraventricular haemorrhage (delicate vessels)
— infection (immature immune system)
— hypoglycaemia

The recognition that low birthweight was sometimes due to

IUGR rather than prematurity was a landmark in perinatal medicine.

The small-for-dates (SFD) infant

1. The baby's weight is below the 10th centile (for that population) for its gestational age. The gestation estimated by dates and scan can be confirmed ($\pm$ 2 weeks) by a detailed neurological and physical examination of the baby.

Growth retardation is usually due to placental insufficiency, but the baby may be small due to congenital abnormality (10%) or infection (CMV, rubella), and these must be excluded.

2. The baby is usually thin, long, with wrinkled skin due to protein-energy deprivation, and has meconium staining of skin, nails and cord due to fetal distress. Such babies are often pink, due to polycythemia (PVC > 70), secondary to intrauterine hypoxia. Unless ill, they feed competently and have little physiological weight loss.

N.B. This classic picture is rare now due to fetal monitoring.

3. The growth-retarded fetus has an increased chance of intrauterine or intrapartum asphyxia. Hypoxia causes the passage of meconium and fetal gasping, hence the tendency to meconium aspiration. There is an increased neonatal mortality rate due to:

— meconium aspiration
— hypoglycaemia (decreased hepatic glycogen)
— polycythemia (jaundice, thrombosis)
— hypothermia (loss of subcutaneous fat)

Management includes aspiration of meconium from the trachea under direct vision at birth, and also gastric aspiration to prevent the meconium aspiration syndrome, and 8-hourly Dextrostix for 3 days.

Neonatal jaundice

The danger of neonatal jaundice is that the high levels of un-conjugated bilirubin can cause kernicterus (the baby becomes irritable and hypertonic) with subsequent retardation, spasticity and high tone deafness.

Any severely jaundiced infant must have serial bilirubin estimation. An increased fluid intake and phototherapy control the serum bilirubin level in most cases. If the bilirubin rises above 350 μmol/l (20 mg/dl), then exchange transfusion may be necessary. The danger level is lower if the infant is pre-term, or if hypoxia, asphyxia or hypo-albuminaemia is present. (e.g. a sick premature baby would have an exchange transfusion above 200 μmol/l)

Day 1   — haemolytic
Day 2-3 — physiological
Day 4   — infection
Day 10   — prolonged

1. Haemolytic jaundice   This develops early because bilirubin is no longer removed by the placenta. Any baby that is jaundiced on Day 1 must be tested for:

— Hb
— group (mother and infant)
— Coombs test
— serial bilirubins

Coombs-positive haemolysis is due to Rhesus incompatibility, or more commonly ABO incompatibility (mother O, baby A), which is usually mild. (Coombs-negative haemolysis is due to spherocytosis or G6PD deficiency, but these usually present after Day 1.)

2. Physiological jaundice   This condition affects 50% of babies and is due to low glucuronyl transferase levels. It develops on Day 2 or 3, peaks around Day 5, does not rise above 200 μmol/l and is gone by Day 10. The baby is completely well.

Bilirubin may rise dangerously high, however, if the baby is preterm or red cell breakdown is increased (e.g. polycythemia, extensive bruising, cephalhaematoma). *Admit if unwell* or bilirubin is above 250 mmol/l (15 mg/dl) on a dermal icterometer.

3. Infection   Infection, especially a UTI, must be excluded if jaundice develops after Day 3 or if the baby becomes unwell:

— MSU
— blood cultures
— chest X-ray
— lumbar puncture
— swabs (umbilicus, throat, stools)

4. Prolonged jaundice   Prolonged jaundice (after Day 10) in a well baby who is entirely breast-fed is usually *breast milk jaundice*. It can last for several weeks. It is harmless and, provided the baby is well, can be ignored. Always exclude *hypothyroidism*, which classically presents with prolonged jaundice (TSH is often screened with the Guthrie test now). In the other causes of prolonged jaundice the baby is usually unwell.

— UTI
— galactosaemia (urine clinitest positive)
— spherocytosis (splenomegaly)
— biliary atresia (steatorrhoea)

Send blood for a blood count and bilirubin (conjugated and unconjugated) and urine for culture and reducing substances.

Hepatitis (due to rubella, CMV, toxoplasmosis α^1-antitrypsin deficiency or idiopathic) and *biliary atresia* both cause a raised conjugated bilirubin (hence there is no danger of kernicterus) with deep jaundice and pale stools, usually developing around the third week. Laparotomy, liver biopsy and cholangiogram are needed to differentiate them.

Vomiting   1. Regurgitation (a feeding problem)
2. Infection
3. Intestinal obstruction
4. Pyloric stenosis
5. Raised ICP
6. CAH
7. Hiatus hernia
8. NEC

1. *Regurgitation.* Most babies regurgitate some milk and air after feeds (*'possetting'*). This can be troublesome if the baby swallows a lot of air with the feeds. This may be due to the hole in the teat being too small or to rapid initial let-down from the breast, or simply to a greedy baby. Adequate winding and larger or more frequent feeds may be required.

2. *Infection* must be excluded in any baby who is vomiting (MSU, swabs, blood cultures, LP). If diarrhoea develops, the diagnosis is probably gastroenteritis.

3. *Intestinal obstruction.* Any baby with *bile-stained vomiting* has intestinal obstruction and should see a surgeon within the hour. There is usually abdominal distension. An inguinal hernia can strangulate easily in the neonatal period and is easily overlooked. *Always examine the groins of a vomiting baby.*

4. *Pyloric stenosis* usually presents between 3 and 6 weeks but can present earlier. Diagnosed by a testfeed, i.e. feeling for a pyloric 'tumour' (like the tip of the nose) during a feed. Treated by pyloromyotomy under local or general anaesthesia.

5. *Raised ICP.* Ultrasound or CT scans may be necessary if irritability, drowsiness, tense fontanelle or fits suggest cerebral or *subdural haemorrhage*. Subdural haematomas can be tapped.

6. *The adrenogenital syndrome* is suspected by virilization in girls, but in boys it presents around Day 7 with vomiting. There is hyponatraemia and serum potassium is high (usually low in vomiting). It is diagnosed by a raised serum 17-OH progesterone level. It is treated with cortisone. It is essential to make a firm diagnosis before starting steroids.

7. *Hiatus hernia* is diagnosed by a barium swallow after the above causes are excluded. The baby is nursed head-up on a tilted surface.

8. *Necrotizing entercolitis* (NEC) is classically seen in preterm infants with an umbilical artery catheter, but can occur rarely in term infants. Mesenteric thrombosis causes gut necrosis and secondary infection, with abdominal distension, vomiting, and malaena. Abdominal X-ray shows air in the gut wall. Treatment involves i.v. fluids, antibiotics and bowel resection. Mortality is 25%.

9. *Haemorrhagic disease of the newborn* can cause blood-stained

vomiting, usually between Days 2 and 4, 1 mg of vitamin K, i.m., is given immediately and blood is transfused. There may also be some blood in the vomit in:

— tube feeding
— cracked nipple (maternal Hb)
— hiatus hernia

In summary, a detailed history is often diagnostic, but the following may be necessary:

— infection screen
— U and E
— test feed
— abdominal X-ray
— barium swallow
— ultrasound or CT scan

Diarrhoea   — gastroenteritis
— infection (UTI, septicaemia)
— drugs (antibiotics, iron)
— (rare: cystic fibrosis, thyrotoxicosis, CAH)

Diarrhoea means frequent watery stools (that may even be mistaken for urine). Dangerous *dehydration can occur within hours*. Signs of dehydration are: loss of skin turgor, sunken eyes and fontanelle, no urine for 6 hours and weight loss.

Breast-fed infants may pass loose green stools with mucus every hour or so at first, as lactation gets established around Day 4–5, but they 'never' get gastroenteritis.

Management   1. Barrier nurse. Stools can be sent for electron microscopy (85% due to rotavirus) and culture (15% due to *E. coli*). Urine should be sent for culture.

2. Stop milk and give 150 ml/kg per 24 hours of a glucose-electrolyte mixture (e.g. Dioralyte) until the diarrhoea stops. Hourly feeds can be tried if there is only occasional vomiting. Once the diarrhoea is controlled, milk is gradually re-introduced, quarter-strength for several feeds and if the diarrhoea does not recur then half-strength, etc (*regrading* the feeds). *Drugs such as kaolin or Lomotil are unnecessary and can be dangerous.*

3. If there is persistent vomiting, the baby has to be admitted for i.v. fluids and U and E monitoring. Admit also if dehydrated or diarrhoea relapses.

4. Recurrence of diarrhoea is usually due to too rapid regrading of feeds, but may be due to secondary *lactose intolerance*, when the stools are Clinitest-positive. It can be confirmed by sending the stools for sugar chromatography. Lactose-free milk may be necessary for several months (e.g. Nutramigen).

5. *Having excluded other causes, the possibility of cow's milk*

allergy is usually considered, and the baby is tired on a soya-based preparation (e.g. Prosobee).

Constipation

Provided there is no difficulty or distress in passing a stool, *the frequency of defaecation is not important*. Some breast-fed babies only pass a stool every 4–5 days. If the stool is hard and painful, increasing the baby's water intake or adding half a teaspoon of sugar to each feed may suffice. If not, a daily glycerine or bisacodyl (Dulcolax) suppository will soften the stool. In severe persistent constipation consider:

— Hirschsprung's disease
— hypothyroidism
— hypercalcaemia
— polyuria (diabetes, insipidus, renal tubular acidosis, salt-losing CAH)

Dyspnoea

— RDS
— pneumonia ($\pm$ aspiration)
— pneumothorax
— diaphragmatic hernia
— congenital lobar emphysema
— choanal stenosis
— congenital heart disease
— severe anaemia

Most of the above can be differentiated on a CXR.

Pneumonia is likely if the membranes were ruptured for more than 24 hours. It may follow meconium aspiration or, in a pre-term baby, aspiration of regurgitated milk.

Tension pneumothorax requires a chest drain and should be suspected in any baby that 'goes off'. Small, asymptomatic pneumothoraces are not uncommon in babies for a few days after delivery.

Diaphragmatic hernias large enough to present as dyspnoea require immediate gastric aspiration, endotracheal intubation and urgent repair.

Congenital lobar emphysema (very rare) is over-distension of one lobe due to an abnormal bronchus acting as a valve, and requires urgent lobectomy.

Choanal stenosis is posterior nasal obstruction. The baby has a submandibular recession as it tries to mouth-breathe, and an oropharyngeal airway produces immediate relief.

Congenital heart disease. A large liver or weight gain suggests heart disease, and an ECG is necessary. If the baby is pale, check the Hb, as a blood transfusion may be life-saving.

Respiratory distress syndrome (RDS)

RDS is likely to occur if the L:S ratio is below 1.5. It is due to deficient surfactant. It affects 50% of babies under 27 weeks and is more common in infants of diabetic mothers. The signs appear within 3 hours of birth.

— tachypnoea
— recession
— expiratory grunt
— cyanosis (later)

CXR may show a ground glass appearance with an air bronchogram, but its main use is to exclude other causes of dyspnoea. *Treatment* involves:

1. Oxygen given by continuous positive airways pressure (CPAP) via a nasal prong, face mask or endotracheal tube. The CPAP prevents the collapse of the alveoli during expiration.

2. Oxygen is monitored by transcutaneous or intra-arterial oxygen electrode, and kept between 6.7 and 12.0 kPa (retrolental fibroplasia)

3. Ventilation is needed if the Po_2 falls despite CPAP or if apnoeic attacks develop. There is a tendency now to early ventilation, especially for LBW babies, and to use CPAP via the endotracheal tube to wean off the ventilator.

4. Fluid balance is monitored. A metabolic acidosis can occur due to poor perfusion, and i.v. bicarbonate may be necessary.

5. Intravenous fluids may be needed for severe dyspnoea, but often the baby can be fed via a nasogastric tube.

6. Antibiotics may be given because the differentiation of RDS and pneumonia (especially due to group B streptococcus) can be difficult.

7. There is some evidence that synthetic surfactant administered via the endotracheal tube improves survival.

Convulsions
— hypoglycaemia
— hypocalcaemia
— meningitis
— cerebral oedema (or haemorrhage)

1. Suck out the pharynx, lay the baby on its side, give oxygen and if still fitting give i.m. paraldehyde (0.2 mg/kg) or rectal valium (0.25 mg/kg).

2. Dextrostix. Hypoglycaemia — defined as blood glucose of less than 1.1 mmol/l — can cause brain damage. If suspected, take blood for glucose and give i.v. 20% dextrose (2 ml/kg), then continuous intragastric milk.

3. If plasma calcium is below 1.8 mmol/l with a normal dextrostix, then 1–2 ml of 10% calcium gluconate is added to each feed.

4. If glucose and calcium are normal, meningitis must be excluded.

5. Phenytoin is given for 48 hours if fits follow birth asphyxia

and trauma. Ultrasound scan may be indicated to diagnose intracranial haemorrhage.

Hypothermia   Hypothermia is a persistent rectal temperature below 35°C and can be fatal. It still occurs in the newborn, especially in LBW babies discharged home to poor conditions in cold weather. *The signs are*:

— weak cry
— poor sucking
— slow reaction to handling
— cold, red skin
— twitching
— oedema (hands and feet)
— sclerema (hardening of subcutateous tissue)

It may causes hypoglycaemia, uraemia, cerebral damage and death.

The baby should be admitted in an incubator for re-warming and biochemical monitoring.

In a cold environment, bonnet, bootees and mittens will help a term infant to retain heat, but a small baby with a low metabolic capacity needs an environmental temperature of at least 27°C (80°F).

Hints for passing the DRCOG

The examination demands a knowledge of:

— obstetrics, with particular emphasis on antenatal care
— postnatal care of mother and child, including resuscitation and examination of the newborn
— all aspects of family planning
— those aspects of gynaecology necessary to the practice of a general practitioner, including cervical cytology

The examination is in three parts:

— written
— clinical
— oral

The written

The written examination consists of four essay questions to be answered in 3 hours.

All doctors are already well qualified to hold their own opinions about sitting examinations, but I feel that the following points are worth making:

The DRCOG is one of the few medical examinations left that requires written essays. The possible topics are quite limited, which is helpful for revision, but having only four essays means that the whole syllabus must be revised, because one very poor essay could fail you.

The DRCOG has the reputation for being a fair and straightforward examination, but people do fail, and failing an easy examination feels much worse than failing a difficult one!

Prepare skeleton essays on the major topics that are likely to come up:

Amenorrhoea	Diabetes	Routine postnatal care
Dysmenorrhoea	Rhesus disease	DVT
Irregular bleeding	Rubella	Resuscitation of the newborn
Infertility	Anaemia	Examination of the newborn
Habitual abortion	Vomiting	Routine care of the newborn
Therapeutic abortion	Abdominal pain	Neonatal jaundice
Pruritus vulvae	APH	Breast-feeding
Vaginal discharge	Unstable lie	Etc.
Cervical cytology	Breech	
Carcinoma of the cervix	Twins	
The menopause	Shared care	
The pill	Criteria for home delivery	
The IUCD	Premature labour	
Sterilization	Induction of labour	
Venereal diseases	Pain relief in labour	
Antenatal monitoring	Delay in the second stage	
Placental insufficiency	Management of the third stage	
Pre-eclampsia	PPH	

Answering an essay usually involves slightly more than regurgitating facts; e.g. instead of 'Write about pre-eclampsia' the question is more likely to be 'Discuss the significance of proteinuria in pregnancy'; or it may involve drawing on information from various subjects, e.g. 'How may perinatal mortality be reduced?' For each subject think up two or three likely essay questions. Some of the sections in this book are intended to provide a framework for essays.

Practise sitting down and writing a formal 45-minute essay at least once before the examination. It takes a surprising amount of self-discipline. Having to sit down and write solidly for 3 hours comes as a nasty shock (high-fliers suck Slow sodium to stave off the writer's cramp).

This may be the first time since Finals that you have had to learn intensively, and even your revision technique may need revision. Also, you now have a full-time job and less time for study, so the following well-known learning techniques are worth bearing in mind:

Before reading a new subject, spend 5 minutes recalling what you already know about it. This takes self-discipline, but is probably the single most useful technique in learning, because it provides a framework for understanding and remembering new facts. Memorizing is most effective when new facts can be linked to current memory (by means of key words).

Diagrams, together with written notes can have a synergistic learning effect. The brain remembers patterns.

Learning is most efficient in bursts of about 40 minutes followed by a rest of at least 10 minutes. Don't waste time struggling over one unclear sentence — make a note of it. It will almost certainly become clear by the time you have covered the subject.

The most efficient way of committing new information to your long-term memory is to recall it. Following an intensive 40 minutes of study the optimum time to recall the material is at:

10 minutes (spend 10 minutes)
24 hours (spend 4 minutes)
1 week (spend 2 minutes)
1 month (spend 2 minutes)
(then every 3 months)

The clinical

The clinical is always an obstetric case. You have about 20 minutes to take a history and to examine the patient (which may include testing a specimen of urine). The clinical part of the examination is usually straightforward, but the following points are worth making:

Routine antenatal clinics do not provide very good practice at taking a full obstetric history so it is worthwhile going to a few booking clinics to see patients before the clinical examination.

The section in this book 'The Obstetric History' includes all the necessary details for a full history and should be memorized.

However, you are not judged on your ability to take a full and detailed obstetric history, but on how you present the case. It is taking an unnecessary risk to go into the clinical examination without having practised some case presentations. Arrange some time with a colleague (preferably senior) to practise presenting a case. It will improve your performance in the examination dramatically.

When you are given the name of your patient write it down (a clipboard and paper are provided); this avoids having to introduce yourself to the patient by saying 'I'm sorry, I've forgotten your name' or having to start off your presentation with 'Mrs err, umm . . .'

Despite any exam nerves, remember to be polite and introduce yourself to the patient before asking when her last period occurred. If she decides she doesn't like you, things may get very difficult.

Jot down the main headings for the history at the left of the page so that you don't miss anything out. Write down positive points but not negative ones. The history may be quite complicated, but take your time and get it all clear. If you take too long and the examiners arrive before you have finished they will give you a bit of extra time and you will not be penalized, whereas if you get the history wrong you will not be forgiven!

You examine the patient twice, once after you have taken the history and once again (briefly) for the examiners.

Remember to take the BP and briefly examine the heart and lungs before turning to the abdomen. Look for scars (particularly laparoscopy scars which can be missed). Decide whether fundal height is compatible with dates and decide on presentation (cephalic, breech or transverse). Listen for the fetal heart and examine for pretibial oedema.

During the examination always continue the conversation because important further information often emerges ('Is the baby still upside down, doctor?'), and it also helps to get the history clear in your mind.

Having examined the patient, always recap on the history and ask in detail about her management. Usually the patient is more than happy to tell you about what has been happening to her, and it helps enormously when the examiner says 'and how would you manage the case?'.

Ask to test a specimen of the patient's urine; (there may not be any available but at least you have asked). It is a simple matter to dip a Multistix into urine and compare the colour on the stick with the colour code on the bottle. However there may be sugar, protein or blood present, so have it clear in your mind how you would manage such findings.

You should have a few minutes spare time between seeing the patient and returning with the examiners. Use the time to get the history in order, to compose a summary and to decide on your management.

There are two examiners (usually one asks questions and the other listens). Good case presentation involves certain simple techniques.

First of all, start off well and have your first sentence well rehearsed ('Mrs Smith is 32 and is expecting her second baby, and she is now 30 weeks by dates and an early scan').

Speak more loudly and more clearly and slowly than normal and make a point of looking up at the examiner every so often to counteract the powerful tendency to mutter and mumble into your notes.

Keep your presentation short — the examiners have heard it all before and won't be paying much attention anyway. At the end of the history they usually say 'Would you like to summarize the history?' and you should have the summary well rehearsed (e.g. 'In summary, Mrs Smith is a Para 2+0 now 30 weeks pregnant by dates and scan; she has been diabetic for 8 years and is presently well-controlled on a BD regime of Retard insulin; she had had no complications until an episode of vaginal bleeding a week ago, when she was admitted and had an ultrasound scan').

The examiner will then ask more details about the history e.g. 'What did you say the birthweight of her previous child was? What other family history did you ask about? Who is looking after the other child at the moment? etc. etc.

The advantage of keeping the presentation brief (despite taking a detailed history) is that the important points are emphasized, the examiner does not get bored and is left with plenty of questions to ask and finally it looks good when he asks you whether you enquired about the patient's social situation (hoping to catch you out) and you are able to give chapter and verse.

Next the examiner will say 'Please show us how you examined the patient.' This simply involves doing what you have done many times before in the antenatal clinic.

He will ask whether you took the BP but will not expect you to take it again, and he will ask questions as you examine the patient ('Why are you doing that?' etc.)

Finally, he will ask some questions about management and the rule is the same as for the viva — answer the question and talk simple common medical sense.

When you have finished it is polite to thank the patient.

The oral

This is the most difficult and most underrated part of the examination. People commonly revise very hard for the written and yet fail to do any preparation at all for the oral section.

Practise 'talking the language' with a colleague who is also preparing for the DRCOG. Prepare a list of four topics each (the maximum for any viva) and arrange a session of about an hour when you viva each other (if there is an audience it adds to the authenticity of the ordeal).

Oral examinations are a good (if random) test of factual knowledge, because you have to understand a subject quite well to be able to talk instantaneously about it. The examiners (usually two, sometimes three) can ask you anything — which is one reason for the fairly detailed notes in this book on neonatal medicine, because most candidates feel obliged to read around the syllabus in order to feel well-prepared and confident.

In oral examinations, however, technique is much more important than knowledge. Most people who fail this section could have talked sensibly about the topics requested — and yet they did not.

There are certain simple techniques concerning oral examinations which can be practised and improved:

Firstly, remember that examiners are only human; the candidate, however knowledgable, is tempting fate if he appears to be untidy, sullen, impolite, hesitant, opinionated or argumentative.

First impressions are very important. The ideal is to appear clean and tidy, to look the examiners in the eye, raise both eyebrows to half-mast, meaning a greeting (any higher may be mistaken for surprise that, perhaps, the examiner does not appear European) give a slight nod and a quick smile (which is different from a grin, a grimace, a smirk or a sycophantic leer) and wait to be asked to sit down.

These comments are not meant to be facetious. We judge and pigeonhole other people within seconds of meeting them. If you keep your eyes glued to the carpet so the examiners cannot see your worried face, or keep your hands in your pockets in the mistaken belief it makes you appear relaxed and in control, you are already doing damage to your cause.

The jargon for this is non-verbal communication, but the fact is you send powerful social signals about yourself (often received unconsciously) even as you walk in and sit down.

Accept the proffered chair, sit halfway between the back and the edge, put both hands together on your knees (so you can't wave them about) and look at the examiners with an air of enthusiasm and humility (it sounds sickening — but these are the rules).

When asked a question, nod slightly as the examiner speaks (rather than making 'not-that-subject' gestures with your mouth) and answer immediately without first saying 'Err'.

Never repeat the question, because it implies that the examiner is being stupid ('You want to know how many cells there are on the average cervix?').

Talk in simple terms about the subject and answer the question. All you have to do is keep talking common medical sense and they are compelled to pass you.

This rule applies particularly to topics that you may feel you haven't covered in enough depth (and there will be at least one). You will still be able to say plenty that is correct and basic, even if it is not particularly original.

If the question is such that you really cannot say anything ('What do you know about the histology of sarcoma botryoides?'), it is best to confess total ignorance immediately, and the examiners will pass straight on to another topic on which you can go on scoring points.

Similarly, if you are at all confused about the question simply ask the examiner to repeat it. It is dangerous to spend five valuable minutes talking rubbish.

If the examiners start their own discussion (or argument) about a particular point, or decide to use your viva time to educate you about their own pet theories — let them! Be interested and don't feel you have to interrupt to get noticed. The cardinal rule of the viva is to get to the end without saying anything stupid.

Never make jokes. The examiner may have a sense of humour but he will not be expecting wit and repartee in a viva; a comment that you intended to be facetious or amusing may get taken seriously ('Well, you see, what I really meant was . . .').

Never ask questions — they are the shovel with which you dig your own grave ('Are you, by any chance, referring to that article in that Swedish journal by Professor Thingummyjig on this sort of thing?' or again 'Do you mean all ovarian tumours or just certain ones?').

Keep off small-print subjects, and certainly never start an answer with small-print — it smacks of little clinical experience ('Amenorrhoea . . . now let me see, well she could have XO/XX mosaicism . . .').

The corollary of this rule is never to introduce a subject about which you know nothing. Examiners are usually helpful, but this includes helping you to construct your place of rest ('All right, tell us about mosaicism.').

Practise doing mock vivas with a colleague and ask him to point out whenever you are breaking the rules ('don't say um, don't repeat the question, don't ask me questions, talk about the subject I gave you, don't start with small-print, don't argue, etc.').

Requirements for entry

The current examination is held twice a year (May and November), and the requirements for entry are:

a) Full registration
b) Proof (a typed statement signed by your consultant) of having held a 'recognized' 6-month appointment either in Obstetrics (when you must also attend ten gynaecology out-patients sessions) or in Obstetrics and Gynaecology.
c) Attendance at eight Family Planning clinics.
d) A fee (which is keeping pace with inflation!)

The diploma examination can only be attempted five times. The Examination Regulations and copies of past papers are available from RCOG. For full details, write to:

The Examination Secretary
Royal College of Obstetricians and Gynaecologists
27 Sussex Place
LONDON NW1 4RG
Telephone 01-262 5425

The Regulations outline the areas of knowledge expected which include:

— Gynaecology
— Psycho-sexual problems
— Sexually transmitted diseases
— Family planning
— Pre-pregnancy counselling
— Antenatal care
— Intranatal care
— Routine examination of the newborn
— Development and Diseases of the newborn

The Regulations also state:

'It will therefore be appropriate for any aspect related to these defined objectives to be covered in the various parts of the examination, but it does not preclude examiners from discussing other topics which are relevant to general practice.'

Glossary of Abbreviations

ACTH	Adrenocorticotrophin
AFP	Alphafetoprotein
AID	Artificial insemination by donor
AIDS	Acquired Immune Deficiency Syndrome
AIH	Artificial insemination by husband
ARC	AIDS-related Complex
AP	Antero-posterior
APH	Antepartum haemorrhage
ASD	Atrial septal defect
BD	Twice a day (*bis in die*)
BP	Blood pressure
BPD	Biparietal diameter
BSO	Bilateral salpingo-oophorectomy
BTC	Basal temperature chart
CAH	Congenital adrenal hyperplasia
CDH	Congenital dislocation of the hip
CIN	Cervical intraepithelial neoplasia
CMV	Cytomegalovirus
CMO	Chief Medical Officer
CPAP	Continuous positive airways pressure
CSF	Cerobrospinal fluid
CT	Computerized tomography
CTG	Cardiotocograph
CVP	Central venous pressure
CXR	Chest X-ray
DHSS	Department of Health and Social Security
DIC	Disseminated intravascular coagulation
DNA	Deoxyribose nucleic acid
DRCOG	Diploma of the Royal College of Obstetricians and Gynaecologists
DVT	Deep vein thrombosis
ECG	Electrocardiogram
EDD	Estimated date of delivery
EE	Ethinyloestradiol
ERPOC	Evacuation of retained products of conception
ESR	Erythrocyte sedimentation rate
ET	Embryo transfer
EUA	Examination under anaesthetic

FBS	Fetal blood sample
FDP	Fibrin degradation products
FH	Fetal heart; family history
FIGO	International Federation of Obstetrics and Gynaecology
FPC	Family Practitioner Committee
FSE	Fetal scalp electrode
FSH	Follicle stimulating hormone
FTA	Fluorescent treponemal antibody (test)
GA	General anaesthetic
GnRH	Gonadotrophin releasing hormone
GTT	Glucose tolerance test
GP	General practitioner
GPI	General paralysis of the insane
Hb	Haemoglobin
HbA_{IC}	Glycosylated haemoglobin
HCG	Human chorionic gonadotrophin
HIV	Human immunodeficiency virus
HPF	High power field
HPL	Human placental lactogen
HRT	Hormone replacement therapy
HVH	Herpesvirus hominis
HVS	High vaginal swab
ICP	Intracranial pressure
IgA	Immunoglobulin A
i.m.	Intramuscular(ly)
IPPV	Intermittent positive pressure ventilation
iu	International unit(s)
IUCD	Intra-uterine contraceptive device
IUGR	Intra-uterine growth retardation
i.v.	Intravenous(ly)
IVC	Inferior vena cava
IVF	In vitro fertilization
IVU	Intravenous urogram
KPPT	Kaolin partial thromboplastin time
LBW	Low birth-weight
LGV	Lymphogranuloma venereum
LH	Luteinizing hormone
LHRH	LH releasing hormone
LMP	Last menstrual period
LOA	Left occipito-anterior
LOT	Left occipito-transverse
LP	Lumbar puncture
L:S	Lecithin-sphingomyelin (ratio)
LSCS	Lower segment caesarian section
LVF	Left ventricular failure
LVH	Left ventricular hypertrophy

MCH	Mean cell haemoglobin
MCV	Mean cell volume
MRC	Medical Research Council
MSAFP	Maternal serum alphafetoprotein
MSU	Midstream specimen of urine
NEC	Necrotizing enterocolitis
NHS	National Health Service
NSU	Non-specific urethritis
NTD	Neural tube defect
OA	Occiputo-anterior
OP	Occipito-posterior
PCV	Packed cell volume
PET	Pre-eclampsia (pre-eclampsic toxaemia)
PGL	Progressive generalized lymphadenopathy
PID	Pelvic inflammatory disease
PNM	Perinatal mortality
POP	Progesterone-only pill
POS	Polycystic ovary syndrome
PPH	Postpartum haemorrhage
PR	Per rectal (examination)
PS	Pulmonary stenosis
q.d.s.	Four times a day (*quater die summendum*)
RBC	Red blood corpuscles
RCGP	Royal College of General Practitioners
RDS	Respiratory distress syndrome
SBE	Subacute bacterial endocarditis
SCBU	Special Care Baby Unit
SCJ	Squamo-columnar junction
SEC	Socio-economic class
SFD	Small-for-dates
SHBG	Sex hormone binding globulin
SLE	Systemic lupus erythromatosus
STD	Sexually transmitted disease
SVC	Superior vena cava
t.d.s.	Three times a day (*ter die summendum*)
TIA	Transient ischaemic attack
TIBC	Total iron binding capacity
TPHA	*Treponema pallidum* haemmagglutination (test)
TPR	Temperature, pulse, respiration
TSH	Thyroid stimulating hormone
TUR	Transurethral resection
U & E	Urea and electrolytes
UK	United Kingdom
UTI	Urinary tract infection

VDRL   Venereal Diseases Research Laboratory (test)
VE   Vaginal examination
VMA   Vanillylmandelic acid
VSD   Ventricular septal defect

WBC   White blood corpuscles
WHO   World Health Organization

YS   Year survival (e.g. 5YS)

Index